YOUR BEST LIFE!

22 Switched On Professionals Share Their Best Strategies For Living Your Best Life... Right Now

W&M

YOUR BEST LIFE I

First published in November 2020

W&M Publishing

ISBN 978-1-912774-76-0 ebk

ISBN 978-1-912774-77-7 pbk

Editor: Andrew Priestley, Kate McNeilly

The rights of Jean-Pierre De Villiers, Julia Cameron De Villiers, Susan Routledge, Immie Adshead, Nipun Kathuria, Renata Ivaštinović, Simon Fletcher, Alison Law, Brady George, Angela Fletcher, Francisco Bricio, Yvette L Baker, Gavin J Gallagher, Speranza Holloway, R.G. Wysocki, Steph Robin, Sumaya Alshamsi, Clare Honeyfield, Yvette K Smith, Hana Abdelkhalek, Kate McNeilly and Andrew Priestley to be identified as contributing authors of this work have been asserted in accordance with Sections 77 and 78 of the Copyright Designs and Patents Act, 1988.

A CIP catalogue record for this book is available from the British Library.

Disclaimer: *Your Best Life I* is intended for information and education purposes only. This book does not constitute specific legal, financial, health, clinical or commercial advice unique to your situation.

The views and opinions expressed in this book are those of the authors and do not reflect those of the Publisher and Resellers, who accept no responsibility for loss, damage or injury to persons or their belongings as a direct or indirect result of reading this book.

All people mentioned in case studies have been used with permission, and/or have had names, genders, industries and personal details altered to protect client confidentiality.

Contents

Welcome To Your Best Life

*"One day you will tell your story of how you've overcome
what you are going through now, and it will become
part of someone else's survival guide."*
Unknown.

Stories have the power to change lives and the world. And sharing what we've been through in our life can help others get through whatever they're currently going through in their lives.

Our own stories of the experiences in our life have the ability to inspire life, opportunity and possibility into people. But when it comes to sharing our stories of what we have been through, and how we got through it, it's important that we share it from a place where we're looking back at your challenges, rather than still being in them. It's important our stories are shared from a healthy, inspirational place of healing.

Whatever we have gone through, we have got through and we have grown through. Be grateful for the fact that you have got through those challenges. Think about it, everything you've ever been through... you've survived.

Otherwise you wouldn't be here reading this book.

As a mindset coach and a speaker, I help people turn their stories from adversity into personal power. And I'm proud to be able to share this book with you, which is a compilation of inspirational stories written by my coaching clients and *Best Life MBA* students about how they have turned moments in their life and even their whole life around. I know without any doubt that this book will open your heart, help you change your perception of how you see your own challenges and life and inspire you to start standing on your story with pride and use it to inspire others.

YOUR BEST LIFE is a book full of powerful tools which you can use to turn your life around and start living your best life.

"When you change the way you look at things,
the things you look at change."
Wayne Dyer

Enjoy this inspirational read.

To your best life,

JP

Jean-Pierre De Villiers

The Power Of Forgiveness

Jean-Pierre De Villiers

I was 37 years old, my life was finally going in the right direction as an international speaker, high performance coach and elite plant-based athlete. I was living the life! It wasn't perfect, but it was pretty close to it.

In May 2019, I was cycling down the UK from John O'Groats to Land's End with a friend to keep fit and raise money for charity. One thousand miles in ten days was the goal. On the eighth day, my life changed forever…

We chose a different route that day and ended up on one with many hills. Usually we finished cycling at 7pm each day after 10 to 12 hours on the road, but on that day, we were still cycling at 7pm.

A few minutes after 7pm I was struck by a drunk hit-and-run driver.

My bike was smashed to pieces and I was thrown off the road, down the side of a bank and left for dead. I ended up spending two weeks in intensive care, fighting for my life with broken legs, broken arm, punctured and collapsed lung, with heart and bowel trauma.

I developed post traumatic amnesia. To this day, I don't remember a thing about the accident. Even though I was told I was conscious at times, I don't remember. The first time I started to realise what had happened was well into my second week in intensive care.

I saw the metal rods sticking out of my legs, tubes hanging out of stomach, arms and neck and bandages and scars covering my body. I knew in that moment that I had a choice.

I had a choice to decide what this was going to mean.

Having been a Coach for most of my adult life and having so many self-mastery tools, I knew that the one thing I wasn't going to do was blame the driver and become a victim.

I took full responsibility for where I was. And one of the first things I said was, *It is what it is*. I accepted what had happened and I surrendered to it.

After weeks lying in hospital, I began a long journey of rebuilding and reinventing myself. It took me to physiotherapists, counsellors, meditation retreats, living in silence for two weeks, living with monks in a Shaolin Temple and working with Dr Joe Dispenza, doing advanced meditations and breath work to heal my body and mind.

I also went on a plant medicine journey to learn how to heal myself at a deeper level.

Over that next year of my recovery, I knew that there was one area I really wanted to work on.

When I woke up in hospital, I knew things like this happen to people and some people allow it to define the rest of their life. It's those people who say many years after something happened to them, "*I am the way I am because of...*".

I didn't want *that* to be me. I didn't want to have this accident break me. I wanted it to make me (better) and I was going to do whatever it took to make it happen.

I was willing to heal whatever needed to be healed. I was committed to working on whatever I needed to work on to free myself and turn this around.

One thing I knew… I needed to know whether I had really forgiven the driver who hit me and left me for dead.

Nelson Mandela once said … *having anger and resentment is like drinking poison and expecting it to kill your enemy.*

Anger and resentment destroys us. And I didn't want it to eat at me. I really wanted to forgive the driver. Not just for me, for him too.

During many months of recovery, I kept waiting for updates on the trial. The first trial was in February 2020.

The accused driver turned up intoxicated, was put in a cell for the night to sober up. The next day he pleaded *not guilty!* No one could understand why he did this, but he did.

Like I said after my accident, *It is what it is…* It was what it was.

I didn't let it get to me. I kept reminding myself that no one is born a bad person. I let that go and waited for the second trial in October 2020.

I was asked if I wanted to appear in court and was told that I didn't have to. But I said, "Yes. I'd like to be there." I wanted to see the man accused of striking me with the car.

I drove four hours across the UK to get to Court. I arrived the day before so that I could be relaxed and at ease.

And I got to the courtroom on time. He was not there. Eventually, I heard that he was found by police on a train in a nearby town - and was intoxicated, again.

The Judge ordered police officers to collect the man. Eventually, they brought him back.

As he came into the building, I stood at the entrance... not to confront him, but to feel what came up. I wanted to feel what was within me. Had I healed myself? Had I moved on? Had I truly forgiven the driver? I needed to know.

When they walked him past me, I felt no anger, hatred or resentment. The only thing I felt was empathy.

Eventually, we got into the courtroom. And after a few minutes the Judge made the decision that the man was not in a fit state to be able to make his plea, so they took him to prison. And we waited again.

I changed some of my plans so that I could be there for another day, and the next morning we were back in court again.

This time, I knew I was ready to face him in court. I was ready to forgive him and say it to his face.

This was my opportunity. I was asked if I wanted to read my Victim Statement out in the courtroom or whether I would like the Judge to read it instead.

My initial thought was, "No, I don't need to read it. I got what I came for. I saw the man yesterday. I feel fine."

Thinking about the man and not myself, I realised that I needed to read the speech. I wanted him to hear it.

There are moments in life where just one person saying one thing at one time can have the potential to change a person's life forever... for better or worse. Has that ever happened to you?

I knew that by not reading my speech there was nothing I could do to help this man change his ways. And that by choosing to read it, I might be able to influence him, to better myself.

In my heart, I knew that there was no way I could *not* read the speech. I wanted to let him know that - even though there are consequences and repercussions for what he did to me - I wished him well, and that in time when he got his sentence to use it to heal whatever he needed to heal, so that he could come out a better, stronger man.

We arrived, and because the accused was already in the cell, he arrived with police escort. We got into the courtroom and at last the man pleaded *guilty* on all charges.

Finally, the judge asked me, "Mr De Villiers, I believe you would like to read your Victim Statement? (Yes, that's what it is called).

I said, "Yes, Your Honour".

I was asked to approach the bench.

I stood behind the microphone and pulled it to my face to read my statement. The speech referred to the accused in third person. I mentioned all the things that had happened in my life since the accident, how my business almost went bust, how my career went from soaring to standing still.

I explained how it affected my life, my mental state and even my relationships.

I finished my speech by saying that I wanted the driver to know that I had no ill feelings towards him and that I had forgiven him.

As I was about to finish my speech, I looked over slightly to my right at the defendant and saw that he had his right hand on his chest and his left hand over his mouth, as if in shock.

When I finished my speech I turned to my left to face the Judge and said, "Your Honour, I would like to add something to my speech, please". What I wanted to say wasn't in my written (planned) speech, so I had to get permission from my lawyer, in line with court formalities. I was taken out of the courtroom, while everyone waited.

I told the lawyer what I wanted to say. She said it was allowed, told the Judge and I was given more time. I stood at the bench over the microphone. As I turned to face the defendant himself, I pulled the microphone up to my mouth so that he could hear me and so that I could look him in the eyes.

I said, "Mr. . . . ., I want you to know that I forgive you and that I wish you the best. I believe that everything happens for a reason and I hope you can use this time to heal whatever you need to heal and come out a better man."

When I was finished the defendant stood straight up. He walked towards the front of the witness box and pressed up against the barrier with his hand on his heart and said, "Your Honour, please, can I share something".

Once the permission was given, he shared with me, "Mr. De Villiers, I'm so sorry, I never meant to hurt you. I think about you and your family all the time, I've even called my lawyers three times to ask how you're doing. I'm so sorry for what I did to you. And if I could, I would have it be me rather than you. I'm so sorry".

We were both emotional. It was one of the most powerful moments in my life.

I knew that the man who almost killed me felt lighter as a result of that experience.

Yes, it was emotional. Yes, it was uncomfortable. But it was incredibly freeing.

I am now free. Free to move forward. Free to live my life. And I'm completely free of anger.

Not letting go of your past and what happened to you or who has done wrong is like trying to swim with an anchor round to your ankle. It will become too heavy for you to carry. Eventually, it will pull you down and destroy you.

If you want to live a happy life, a free life… let go.

This includes forgiving yourself.

Let go of your past mistakes.

Let go of your past failures. Just because you have failed, it doesn't mean that you are a failure. Don't label yourself as a failure. Learn from the experiences you've had. Learn from the people who have come your way, whether in good or bad times.

Your past does not have to define your future. You can use your past to create a powerful future. But just like I was faced with a choice when I woke up in intensive care, and I was faced with a choice to attend or not, and I was faced with a choice when asked to read that letter in court. You are responsible for making our own choices... every day.

If you want to live your best life you've got to let go of everything that's holding you down. Not only with this help accelerate you into an extraordinary life in future, but it will remove suffering from your life right now, in the present.

Holding on to anger has no way of serving you. So let it go.

Ask yourself:

- Where do I have anger in my life?

- Who do I need to forgive?

- What do I need to forgive myself for?

I want to share a powerful Hawaiian practice with you. It's called *Ho'oponopono* which is the following mantra:

I'm sorry.

Please forgive me.

Thank you.

I love you.

It will help you embrace forgiveness in your life and repeating this mantra every day will make it easier to start forgiving yourself and to forgive others. You will be the main beneficiary of forgiveness, no mistake.

I promise you, the more you embrace forgiveness in life... the lighter and happier your life will be.

I forgive you. I love you.

About Jean-Pierre De Villiers

Jean-Pierre (JP) is a Transformational Speaker, Performance Coach, Author, Plant-based Athlete and the founder of the Best Life MBA Coaching Community.

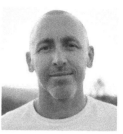

JP coaches people how to tap into their full potential and perform at their best by transforming their body and mind and spirit.

With almost two decades of experience in peak performance and personal coaching, JP is renowned for running transformational events, seminars and challenges globally, stretching people to be their absolute best.

Business leaders, entrepreneurs and artists have benefited from JP's expertise and have relied on him to help them perform at the highest level. JP teaches leading-edge strategies to keep his clients ahead of the game.

As well as speaking internationally and being hired by large global organisations for his high impact coaching skills, JP regularly contributes to publications and features in the media. He is the author of several books, is a professional martial artist, has completed multiple ultra-marathons and other endurance events and is an Ironman triathlete.

JP has shared the stage with some of the world's best speakers including Lisa Nichols, Jay Abraham, Prince EA, Jay Shetty, Robert Kiyosaki and Dr. John Demartini.

www.jeanpierredevilliers.com

Surrender

Julia Cameron De Villiers

I was a creative dreamer as a child. It was the one thing that created excitement, energy and inspiration in my life - and still does. I was always thinking of creative ideas and even at a young age I was quite the entrepreneur.

At around 9 years of age, one of my earliest ventures was turning our playroom into a hotel and inviting friends round to stay as my guests.

At the makeshift reception desk, I would have a large tin of penny sweets that I bought from the newsagent opposite my house. I charged not one but two pence for them, making a penny a piece. I would then reinvest in more stock only to eat most of it myself. Buying one sweet guaranteed your entry for the night which was a bed behind the curtain I had created out of an old trunk. The presidential suite was worth two penny sweets and was an emporium of delights in a cupboard under the main hallway stair. It had pictures of painted rabbits on the wall, a Persian rug and even a little lamp. Really quite luxurious, if I do say so myself.

I absolutely loved it!

And I knew then that as long as I was connecting with people, making them feel good, creating experiences and something that was mine I would be happy and well on my way to leading my best life.

If only I had been as wise during my teens and early twenties.

Having been bullied through school, I stopped believing in the dreams and ideas I had because it seemed that whatever made me inherently me, also made me a target for bullies. I had no self-esteem and started formulating ideas on who I was meant to be based on what I thought would make me more popular. I became a rebel child and started dabbling in drugs and alcohol from a young age which progressed through my teens and into my mid-twenties. I became someone that was totally fueled by a hedonistic lifestyle which eventually lead me to rock bottom. I lost my way so badly that I ended up alienating myself from family, friends and ultimately myself. I didn't know who I was outside of being a *party* person. At my worst, I woke up from a drug- induced stupor on the side of a cliff just inches from certain death.

With no positive influences around me at my lowest point, I didn't think I was ever going to recover. I wasn't looking after my health, I could barely string a sentence together and I had the mental focus of a fish. I kept manifesting situations in my life where I felt trapped because that's how I felt inside. Instead of living for what lit me up like I did as a child, I was living as a lost soul, someone who lived to fit in with what others wanted from me. I didn't know that in life if we want things to change all we have do is make a decision and ask the universe for help, for something better.

I thought I had to do everything on my own.

The night I hit rock bottom, I was living in Spain and felt trapped in a situation where I was working for someone who was abusive and not paying me. I didn't think I had anyone to turn to or anywhere to go.

Again, I was trapped.

I didn't have the confidence to say no or stand up to anyone that was mistreating me. I felt that this was my mess and my mess alone. Mentally and physically unwell due to the lifestyle I was leading, I felt completely lost and couldn't see a way out. I had become hostage to the mental limitations I had placed on myself.

I remember looking at the swimming pool in their garden and wondering if I could drown myself in it but deep down inside I knew that wasn't the way out. I remembered the bright future I had imagined as a child and I knew somehow it was possible for me. I just had to find inner strength.

That night I went for a walk outside, looked up to the skies and called out to God, *Please help me get out of this situation, please help me to find myself and make something of my life.*

It was time for divine intervention.

From that moment on things started to change. I had finally surrendered. I realised I didn't have to accept what is, I had the power to change things.

I started my own jewellery business not long after and was finally inhabiting the fun and creativity that I dreamt of as a child. I was living the dream on the one hand - creating something really exciting, meeting new people, doing photo shoots and having fun - whilst on the other I was still struggling because I never believed I was worthy to receive success. I tended to do things for my ego, so that people would think I was doing great. I needed the admiration so badly because I had no self-esteem. With a lack of self-esteem you tend to have very low boundaries and I would often get myself into sticky situations because I allowed people to take advantage of me or would do things that made no business sense. Luckily during this time, I believe as a response to my call for help from the universe, I started to attract mentors who taught me the value of discipline and self-love. When others invested in me, I started believing in myself again. The healing process continued as I started to fill myself up from within.

I discovered the law of attraction and started implementing its practices right away. I came to know that in life we get what we believe we deserve. I started creatively visualising just as I did as a child and things started showing up for me. The more I said yes to things I enjoyed and started showing up for my health and wellbeing, my life unfolded in ways that I couldn't have imagined.

Soon after, I manifested my husband and started living a life of freedom where I was able to be just who I was! I realised that all I wanted in life was to be creative and look after those I love but it wasn't until I served myself first that I began healing and unlocking what I already always knew in my heart.

Through my journey I've learnt that living your best life is truly an inside job and it starts with self-love and self-worth. Once you have that your life will look very different. You will only accept relationships in your life that lift you up. You'll learn to trust your intuition and flow with the path of your highest calling by following what feels good and letting go of what doesn't.

You see, when we really look at what lit us up as children, there is always a common theme and that thread is what makes up our nature self, the true self, the one that creates for the sake of creating, for the joy of it and not just for the financial reward. Sifting out our true self from the one that has been conditioned over the years to conform or fit what we think we should be doing is the key to unleashing our personal pot of gold. That of our spirit, divine self and the one that already knows how worthy and perfect we are just as we are. That is the key to living a life on purpose that feels fulfilled.

I'm now the happiest I've ever been and that's because I've let go of trying to be something I'm not. I've learnt to embody the concept of surrender. Surrendering to what is and not trying to force life into a shape that's not meant for you is truly liberating and there is nothing more valuable in life than feeling free.

My favourite saying is *It's on its way* because the moments that make up your best life always are.

They just may not come as you expect them to.

About Julia Cameron De Villiers

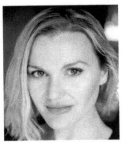

Julia Cameron De Villiers is the visionary behind the JCDV Jewellery Brand where she creates jewellery with soul, incorporating designs with an empowering aesthetic. A multi-expressive creative and people connector known for having her finger on life's pulse, Jules has contributed articles to magazines such as Hip & Healthy, Women's Health and The Incredible Magazine. Her jewellery has been worn by celebrities such as Keira Knightley and featured in Harpers Bazaar. She has spoken on the TedX stage and is the Vice President of Dimbola Museum where she is passionate about sharing the work of her ancestor Julia Margaret Cameron who was a trailblazing creative of the Victorian era that never conformed to the conventionalities of her day.

Jules is an entrepreneur at heart, author, voice-over artist and designer with a passion for wellness, creativity and helping others overcome fear and self doubt so that they can live the kick ass dream life of freedom they deserve and, in the process, become the best version of themselves.

Contact Julia Cameron De Villiers

https://www.instagram.com/jcdvjewellery/

https://www.instagram.com/julescamerondv/?hl=en

www.jcdvjewellery.com

Whose LIFE Are You Living?

Susan Routledge

It may sound a strange question to ask, but I think all to often it can be so easy to be influenced by peers and to end up on a totally different life journey.

All I can ever remember wanting, was to be in the beauty industry.

From being very small I loved the thought of enhancing someone's looks with my hand-me-down cosmetics collection, much to the horror of any visitors (victims!) who came to my home, and then dared to linger for any length of time.

I was really timid as a child, but I was brought up by the perfect parents - for me - within a small town in the North East of England:

My mother, the perfect homemaker truly believed I could be and do anything.

My father, a hard-working foreman joiner by day and

a property developer entrepreneur by night, and every weekend.

They were perfect parents for me, but not together.

As a teenager, my parents divorced, but I saw this as a bonus, not a negative, as I now had dedicated time to spend with my Dad without the family tension and arguments. It was time often spent collecting rents, but it was still quality time to me.

My Dad's plan was to work like crazy, make as many property investments as possible and then to retire early at 55, and live off the profits.

So, the fact that I wanted to go to college to study Beauty Therapy and Hairdressing, which back in the late 1970s was a 4-year course, seemed totally crazy to him.

Beauty jobs were rare, and really low paid. My Dad could never see how there was ever going to be any money working in the beauty industry. The industry was so small back then, hence why all courses combined hairstyling too.

I didn't even know how I could afford to train as the nearest courses were hundreds of miles away... but then, as I was due to leave school, a course opened up in my region and I knew I had to be on it.

I didn't have a clue what I wanted to do by the end. I just thought I would figure that out later, after all I had four years to think about it.

As the course drew to a close, I had increasing pressure from my Dad to find a job, but all of the decent jobs would mean living away.

I was terrified I wouldn't get a job, so I decided my best option was to start a beauty and hairdressing freelancing business without initially telling my Dad.

So, with fliers in hand, my Mum and I spent a full day posting leaflets out, which was by far the cheapest advertising in the early 1980s.

To my total surprise, the hallway telephone was ringing by the time we got back. So, I started the next day, with my car packed and ready to visit my first clients and with my Mum at home as my makeshift receptionist.

I became so busy, so quickly. Word certainly flies around a small town. There were only two things wrong. About 95% of my clients wanted hairdressing services as beauty certainly hadn't caught on in my small town. The other thing was that I was working ridiculous hours as I didn't want to let anyone down, or to turn anyone away.

To start with it didn't matter. I was making great money. My Dad, by now had found out and offered to help me with my book-keeping but I decided to keep it under wraps until I could unequivocally prove to him that I was successful.

I had this vision of sitting him down at the table, opening my amazing accounts book and my Dad being so, so proud.

That day never came.

On an early February night, my Dad went to bed and never woke up again. He was days away from his 51st birthday. He had a huge cerebral haemorrhage which instantly ended his life.

It just didn't seem real. I just couldn't take it in.

I had driven passed my Dad the day before. He was up a ladder and looked busy and I certainly didn't have time to stop as I was racing to my next appointment. I just thought I would see him later, but that day was never to be.

I didn't know what to do. I wanted to just run away, but I had all of my clients to see. Cancelling them just meant a longer wait list, so I did what I thought my Dad would expect me to do and carried on working as much as I could.

I started to resent the business I had created. I resented that it was so demanding. I resented that that I had no free time. I resented that it had stopped me chatting to my Dad on that last day of his life. I resented that I hadn't had chance to show him my accounts book. I resented everything, including that it wasn't even the career that I wanted.

I realised that I just wanted to prove to my Dad I could do it, and now I was trapped in it all.

I now firmly believe that the universe will always correct things, and although no-one could bring my Dad back, I believe that there are external forces helping you.

Within weeks of my Dad's death, I developed a really severe rash all over my hands. I had always protected my hands with gloves whilst working, but this rash came out of the blue and I started reacting to everything associated with hair products.

It was so painful that it would make me cry. I was so low anyway, but just putting this happy face on for the world.

My GP told me that I must look for another career and although it was a relief, I still had so many people relying on me visiting their homes, many who were housebound.

By now this business had no meaning for me and one day I literally gave my whole business away to another stylist.

Over the next couple of years, I took on retail jobs. I just wanted minimum responsibility and time to heal. I stumbled upon a book by Louise Hay called, *You Can Heal Your Life.*

I was fascinated, and this started my never-ending journey in self-development.

By now the Beauty Industry was gaining momentum and I decided to take some refresher courses and start all over again.

This time felt very different though. I had a clear vision and total belief that I was on the right path for ME, and nothing was going to stop me.

I started freelancing again, but this time just in beauty therapy, and also got a position teaching in a private college one day a week.

Within exactly one year, I opened my first small salon. I started employing staff within six months and quickly outgrew this space.

I found my perfect property and bought 50% of the building. I couldn't afford it all, so I persuaded my boyfriend at the time to buy the other half until I could afford to buy, and then expanded over the next building.

Soon we were the largest Beauty Salon in my region and one of the largest in the UK.

I used to constantly dream and focus on what I wanted next. I would write myself notes of what seemed outrageous at the time.

I always believe that if someone else has done it, then I can do it too.

I made myself a note declaring that my salon would win the *National Title of Best UK Beauty Salon*. It was a really big ask as previous winners were city centre salons and my business was 14 miles from any city. We won the title on our second attempt.

This was the start of over 12 *National Business Awards*.

I have always created amazing teams around me, and I systemised the business to work independently of me.

I stepped out of the business and I have the pleasure of working as a global business consultant, international speaker, Awards Judge, industry advisor and totally passionate with all I do. I am blessed to attract the best clients and the most amazing network of people to work with.

Along my journey I created my own formula for creating my best life on an analogy of L.I.F.E which I would love to share with you.

- **The L is for LOVE.** I always aim to only do what I love. I send love daily to myself plus everyone and everything. In return I only attract the best people to me, without fail.

- **The I is for INVEST.** I invest time and energy in myself on a daily basis. I meditate every day and spend time journaling, reading and visualising what I want to create. I have a never-ending thirst for personal development.

- **The F is for FOCUS.** I only focus forwards and in a positive way. I believe everything happens for a reason, giving us emotional feedback and an opportunity to think better thoughts. I don't ever dwell in negativity as it keeps us stuck and attracts more of the same.

- **The E is for EXPECT.** This is a huge one. You can only create what you truly believe and expect to happen.

As I previously said, "I believe that I can create anything that anyone else has achieved", and you can too. My true wish for you, is to live your Best Life created by yourself, for yourself.

About Susan Routledge

Susan Routledge is a Multi Award Winning Salon Owner and Global Business Consultant. She specializes in creating cash rich businesses, which give the business owner ultimate freedom, plus the tools and support to develop themselves outside of their business too.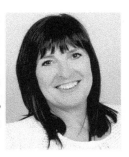

Susan helps her clients to find hidden untapped revenue streams, whilst building and maintaining a totally loyal clientele and highly motivated team.

She is the founder of her trademarked STABLE business formula, plus a sought-after Business Turnaround Consultant and author of *The Little Book of Client Retention*.

Her down to earth, light-hearted approach has made her a trusted Industry Advisor, International Speaker and Awards Judge.

Susan's online blog, *Beauty Entrepreneurs,* has attracted over 7,000 global subscribers for her weekly hints, tips and insights. She also has an online business turnaround programme called *Salon Success Freedom* and is the creator of *Beauty Directors Club*, a monthly membership for salon business resources and advice.

Contact Susan Routledge

http://susanroutledge.com

http://beautydirectorsclub.com

The Power Of
The Movement Mindset

Immie Adshead

WARNING: *Building a strong movement mindset can set off an unstoppable chain reaction of redefining your perceived limits beyond what you can fathom...*

Lining up shoulder to shoulder, waist deep in the cool lake water with bare feet sinking down into the squidgy mud below. The silence and suspense running down the start line, then BANG! The start gun fires, the adrenaline pumps, the melee of limbs kicking and splashing. Months of anticipation, hours of training and focus coming down to this moment. The moment where it's you versus you. A 1500m swim, 40km bike and 10km run lies between you and the finish line, where you'll break through the barriers of possibility and redefine what's possible.

Sport has always been part of my life and I'm fortunate to work as a fitness coach, specialising in the body-brain connection.

I'm able to show my clients a movement mindset and inspire them to do the same. One of the most powerful moments that sport has given me is from competing in triathlons. I've experienced and competed in many different sports and I loved (almost) every moment of them! I've noticed that throughout my life to date, the points where I've felt most in flow are when I've had a sport to train and compete in, with the support of the community within a team or club.

At the start line of the Hever Castle Triathlon Olympic distance race something was different: compared to previous experiences this was the catalyst for something much bigger. If you'd told me that I'd be completing an Ironman in just less than a year from then I'd not have believed it.

An Ironman distance is 3800m swim, 180km bike and 42.2km run. By the time I crossed the finish line at Hever Castle, I had achieved what had seemed impossible. In fact, I was hungry for a bigger challenge! Boundaries are merely ideas constructed in our minds and we can choose where they go!

To work with clients to redefine those boundaries around fitness is the most rewarding part of my coaching. The power of it is huge. One of the biggest breakthroughs has been working with a client who found walking 1km challenging. We set an aim to walk 5km as part of an organised race two months into our training programme. Of course, the goal was achieved. My client subsequently has walked the 5km distance many times. The movement mindset can be redefined from any position. We all have our boundaries set to different configurations. No configuration is better than the other, the important part is to reconfigure them to expand our possibilities.

To add some context before racing at Hever Castle (in Kent, UK), I had been living in Dubai, UAE, setting up my fitness coaching business for roughly two years since 2017. I had become so focussed on building a successful business that I had forgotten to focus on my own fitness and have a goal to work towards myself. I tried different sports but none of them inspired me to level up.

To be truly living to your full potential you should be leading by your actions, not just your words. After all people copy what you do, not what you say! I can safely say that I was not doing this at this point. I was letting myself fall short of my full potential both in my business and fitness. Adding a focus gives us purpose: we know the answer to what and where we need focus, but often we need someone to ask the right questions and guide us on a path.

Competing in triathlons not only gave me a focus and a stronger mindset but also a community of like-minded athletes. Never ever underestimate the power of community. As human beings we thrive in them! After all, nothing great is ever achieved alone. We always go further with a community of people behind us. Within these communities powerful friendships can be found that last a lifetime!

2020 has been a challenging year for most. For me it has meant switching my business primarily online, lockdowns and choosing to move back to the UK after almost four years in Dubai (an incredible place with incredible people!) Globally, not the easiest time, but there was one thing that kept me going; an event to focus my training on and a community that had my back.

Training gave me focus throughout the Dubai lockdown, something constant to work towards even when every other part of my life seemed uncertain.

The human body is an intricate machine and there is something that resonates when training or competing. For me it's like an active meditation as you glide through the water between strokes of the swim, feel the lactic acid burn as you power up the hills on your bike or tune in to the beat of your footsteps as you run. In that moment, you are in the present and nothing else matters.

In our modern lifestyle it's easy to get swept up in fretting about the past or the challenges of the future. Training in the triathlon disciplines is a route to keep me in the present. It's a way to stay grounded.

The present is where we are now and that's where we take the steps forward towards our bigger goals. What's the point worrying about the next 10,000 steps when the important one is right now in this moment? Each step may not be perfect, but it takes us one step closer. A workout is a part of the day that you can switch off from anything else happening in your life and be in the now. This is especially important today more than ever with our modern lifestyle.

For me, triathlons were the key that allowed me to shift my mindset up a gear. From my experience, a strong movement mindset where fitness is a non-negotiable is the root that everything stems from. Humans are built to thrive on movement, it resonates with our DNA!

When you understand and implement the dynamics of body-brain connection the results are much more powerful. This is my strategy when working with my clients.

The brain is the CEO of your body and acts as a newsroom with the reporters (eyes, inner ear vestibular system and proprioceptive map stored within your brain) feeding in information for your brain to base decisions on. The better the quality of information from the reporters, the better the decisions you make.

This is seen most effectively with the eyes and posture.

Our eyes lead our bodies, so when you look down it is easier to hunch over. The optimal information to stand taller is a view of straight ahead. By just changing the eyes we change how we stand. If you want to stand taller right now look straight ahead, try it as you walk. Please make sure you still look where you're going though!

The power of understanding the whole system not only allows you to change posture more effectively, but also how to manage injuries and improve movement range.

The brain's job is to keep you alive, it will protect you from any perceived threats. It is important to understand from your brain's perspective. An injury is an area that the brain wants to protect. Certain movements may make the brain feel threatened, kicking in the protection instinct of blocking all movement around the injury. By working with the body-brain system we can show that the perceived threat is in fact harmless. Show your brain the pathways that you want to reinforce, and achieve powerful long lasting results by understanding how the whole system interacts. The mind is powerful, so to truly unlock the movement mindset it requires both body and brain.

As with many events this summer the Ironman event I had trained so hard for was cancelled due to the pandemic.

This didn't mean that I couldn't do the event... after all, it is not the event that was the important part. It was the journey and the process of transforming into a stronger, more resilient person. It's never the thing, it's the thing about the thing. The event would be a celebration, a showcase of everything I'd been working towards. I chose to run my own DIY event using a local lake to swim in, the indoor trainer to cycle 180km and a local loop to run a marathon.

Remember we choose where to define the limits!

Triathlon was the key that unlocked the movement mindset for me. It showed me new levels that I never knew existed. I truly believe that a movement mindset can give anyone who wants to find it the ability to break through the barriers that currently hold them back. It doesn't matter what level you start at, the most important thing is the level you are heading towards!

It's not where you start, it's where you finish. Begin today, move more, build your movement mindset and live your best life now!

About Immie Adshead

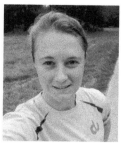

Immie is a L4 personal fitness coach specializing in optimizing the body-brain connection to enable her clients to achieve full fitness potential. She has built a wealth of experience over 6 years in both Dubai and UK. She's worked in partnership with a leading UAE telecoms company enabling a motivated and healthier workforce.

She's now UK based offering online or online/in-person hybrid programmes. Through her in-depth understanding of how the body-brain interacts she is able to optimize results for clients: improving posture, movement patterns and reducing pain.

As an author of multiple ebooks and published co-author she aims to spread awareness of the power of the body-brain approach to fitness coaching. Immie's ultimate goal is to inspire others to adopt a movement mindset with non-negotiable fitness, helping them to achieve their ultimate fitness potential and live their best life.

Immie is a keen triathlete and Iron(wo)man, demonstrating the power of the movement mindset to inspire others.

Contact Immie Adshead

www.thebodybraincoach.com

@the.body.brain.coach

The Ultimate Purpose

Nipun Kathuria

Life is a dance that requires juggling various goals and aspirations simultaneously. Most of us do regular goal setting for various areas of our life: financial, health, relationship or spiritual.

From the outside to me, they always seemed like different goals that resulted in different outcomes. I had a seismic shift in my understanding when I started working on my personal and spiritual development and found that all these outcomes actually led to the same road, which is the road to happiness.

While doing goal setting, most of the life coaches talk about the seven levels deep exercise which is asking yourself seven follow up questions on your initial WHY. This helps you uncover your ultimate WHY.

The first few answers come from the conscious side, while the subsequent answers are deep as they come from your subconscious.

When I tried the same exercise on my financial, health, relationship and spiritual goals, I found that the ultimate

WHY I was going after was happiness. And every single time, this has never failed me.

Go ahead and apply this exercise yourself.

As humans, we all crave for happiness, which is quite ingrained in us. Also to note here is that the cycle of happiness sits on the wheels of balance.

My spiritual master from India constantly stresses balance in life. He says that every object of creation in this world has to maintain balance. All creatures, except humans, maintain a balance in their natural states. He further says that all human beings need to be conscious of balancing their lives. He says that the 24 hours in a day should be enough to balance various areas of your life from career to spirituality. And I have always found this to be true. The source of ultimate happiness is balance.

Now, if we know that happiness is our ultimate purpose in life, how can we achieve that? I have shared below some experiences and learnings that have truly changed my life in the last four years:

Lower Your Expectations (Of Others)

I am an ardent follower of the teachings of Tony Robbins. He always says: *Trade your expectations for appreciations, and your whole life will change.*

Four years ago, when I first heard about this, I found it very superficial. But in the last few years, since I started to implement it, I can clearly see the positive impact such a small way of living can bring to your day to day life. There was a time people used to affect me in a certain way, especially when those who were close to me did not live up to what I expected of them. I spent a lot of my time and energy contemplating this, creating a story in my head and then thinking of reasons why I can't have the same relationship with that person ever again. Now that I think about it, I was immature and foolish perhaps.

Most of the times we do not know the circumstances that resulted in that person behaving a certain way. I used to make a fictional story in my head without knowing the facts and then apologising at the end once I realized the true facts. Haven't we all been there and done that?

My more seasoned self now tries not to jump to conclusions in these scenarios. I always tell myself that everyone has their own priorities and that doesn't make them bad or wrong. I appreciate them for all they have done for me. This allows me to conserve my time and energy. I have found much peace in life by adopting this mindset.

Expect High Standards When It Comes To Your Health

Back in school, I hated biology. I never liked to know how the human body works. I never thought that one day I will be writing about health and how to use your body as a vehicle to achieve that ultimate purpose. I still remember that I used to sit in my room and study, while my friends participated in sports and outdoor activities. I was unapologetic at that time because I thought that if I will do well in my studies and work, it should compensate for all the time not spent on health and fitness. I couldn't have been more wrong.

Four years ago one fine day, it was a regular Sunday and as I tried getting up from my couch, I froze and there it was –

I could not get up. Medical diagnosis revealed a herniated disc or as they commonly call it slipped disc. I was young and had never been in an accident. The only thought that was in my head was — *why me?*

That one incident changed my whole perspective towards health and the importance of maintaining a balance between work and health. I might not have fully recovered, but the last few years have taught me so much about fitness. I feel much younger, more energetic and happier all day, every day.

My wife makes fun of my old pictures of our wedding as I looked so different and heavier then. I now use fitness as a vehicle to achieve goals in other areas of my life. As my coach, Jean Pierre De Villiers would say, *Fitness should be one of your non-negotiables.*

Don't let a physical ailment remind you of how important health is for a happier life.

Getting Uncomfortable

There are times when you feel everything moves slowly, including your life and there are other times when you see tremendous growth.

If I recollect the occasions when I experienced a sudden growth in my career or finances, that was when I became uncomfortable. I was one of the millions of engineers in India, when I decided to invest in my education and move to Ireland. I left my job to study in a country that was ten times more expensive than India.

Tough decision. But now when I look back, it was one of the best that I had ever made. I feel content career wise, and financially, and I am able to now help people which I couldn't have done earlier.

Another tougher decision following that was to leave a comfortable day job to manage the digital team of one of the biggest and fastest growing high street retailers in the UK and Ireland. Looking back now, I owe everything I know about digital and marketing to the world-class mentors I had over the last few years. Because of this exceptional experience, I now run my own company where I help small businesses leverage new opportunities in the digital era. Where I am today, I am much happier and content, although I work much harder than before. I sometimes wonder where I would have been, if I hadn't taken that leap of faith, gotten out of my comfort zone...

Certainty

Humans always look for certainty in things, but we also know that the only constant in life is change. I always found those two principles contradictory.

My spiritual master always said that things happen in our lives for a reason, with the sole purpose to help us grow.

In the last few years, since I have been conscious of this principle, I have started noticing that whenever I am facing problems or if circumstances force me to do certain things, there is always a hidden learning or benefit for me. I used to ignore those cues because I never believed in that principle. The more I practice it now with small things, the more this principle supports me in bigger things in life. The issue with my back that I talked about earlier has been a blessing in disguise for my health. Although it's not ideal to get up each day in pain, it always reminds me the importance of fitness and has helped me be in the best shape I have been in my entire life. This certainty of the higher purpose, has guided me in my life to stay happier by being more patient and having faith that things will work out.

In the end, I would just like to say that one of the scales you should measure your growth in life is on the scale of happiness. Find a friend, a coach, a teacher or a colleague who will help you move forward towards your true purpose. Once you realise that your ultimate purpose is happiness and see yourself growing, life becomes much simpler.

About Nipun Kathuria

Nipun Kathuria is the founder of a leading e-commerce development and digital marketing company in Ireland called *Technik*. Nipun works with small and medium sized businesses, helping them leverage their digital presence. After having led global teams in technology 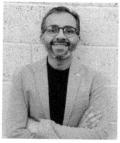 and retail businesses, his mission is to bring these digital resources to small and medium sized businesses. He is well known in the e-commerce and marketing circles in India and Ireland. He also mentors business school graduates and young start-ups. His other mission is to help people lead the best version of their lives.

Although Nipun holds an engineering degree from India and an MBA from Trinity College Dublin, he believes that his real education and expertise is in business and personal development.

He is also a published author, a personal development enthusiast, a marathon runner, a loving son to his parents and a loving husband to his beautiful wife.

Contact Nipun Kathuria

https://linktr.ee/technik

Jump! JUST JUMP! Now!

Renata Ivaštinović

Since I was a child I knew I would do it. But how?

I was standing on the edge of a high building, so high I couldn't even see what was below. I'm falling into darkness. That feeling in my chest was so intense that I woke up. I wondered if it was a dream or reality. After dreaming the same dream several times, I decided: *I will find out how it really feels. I'll jump out of the plane!*

Wise to have a parachute as well, of course!

Why have I decided to share my personal story with you? We all feel fear of something. Fear is one of the strongest emotions. Fear of heights, fear of falling, fear of failing, fear of losing stable ground, fear of losing job, financial fears, fear of unknown, even fear of fear itself…

Today, there's an enormous amount of uncertainty and anxiety and we are going through lot of fear, particularly now in 2020 (at the time of writing this).

How to deal with that in a business environment?

I never considered myself a victim of circumstances. We can feel fear and still take some actions. Fear is just telling us that we should protect and prepare ourselves. This story is about how I faced my fear and jumped with the parachute while, the same year, I was transitioning from a corporate career to entrepreneurship.

How motivated I will be to change what I don't like in my personal or professional life depends on my beliefs and values.

Today I consult, train and coach clients who have lost their jobs, but also those who are not happy with their current work situation. Some of them are not sure if they want to work for someone else and look for a new job or start their own business. I tell them that not all of us need to be entrepreneurs, but we can be more entrepreneurial.

Our behaviours and our environment are easiest to change. Still, I'm not saying that it's easy. Do your activities take you where you say you want to go? How consistent is what you say with what you do, what you are capable of doing and what you believe? Do you allow yourself to do something different from what society, family, friends or the company you work for think you should, want, could, dare?

If not, what is stopping you from doing it?

Through the process we come to our values. It's great if your values and beliefs are aligned with those of the company or people you work with. However, if that is not the case, it can be a problem. You can solve this problem by changing the way you think. Or not, because you may not be willing to change your beliefs and values.

Some people I know left the companies they worked for when their values and integrity became compromised. Although the alternative was uncertainty, they made their choice. I was in the same situation as well.

If you are not sure which way to go, ask yourself:

- *Who are you being in this situation?*

- *What is important to you?*

- *What are your personal values?*

If you are building your own business, you should align your business with them. Find out what drives you. What is your reason to get out of bed and, no matter how you feel, are you committed to achieving your goal?

You can examine that from various sources, i.e. through coaching sessions, mentors, assessment centres, online assessments, peers etc. I took a paper and put a title: *Wonderful Life.* Then I wrote down my pros and cons.

For each opportunity, I thought, *What could possibly go wrong? What is the worst scenario that could happen? What are all good and great things about it?*

Then, I negotiated with myself. If you follow the process, you will probably realize that good things and bad things come in the same package. But at some point you need to decide: *Is this the right package for me? Is it worth taking a risk?*

I was sitting in the office and somehow we started to talk about who is afraid of what. I mentioned that I hadn't jump with the parachute yet, but I was determined to do it. My colleague said that he already jumped, a few times even, as he enrolled in a parachute school that included five parachute jumps. I was so excited and impatient to hear how it was.

Do you want the truth or something beautiful?

Only the truth, please!

During my first jump, I was terrified. From the very first second until we hit the ground, I was so afraid.

Was it better on the second jump? You already knew what to expect.

Not really. I was still very scared.

Well, I guess you've overcome that to the fifth jump?

I didn't even get to the fifth. After the third I gave up!

Never mind! I decided. I will jump! And, when you want something, as Paulo Coelho wrote in *The Alchemist: All the universe conspires in helping you to achieve it.*

There are several ways to get from point A to point B. The experiences of others are literally that – just the experiences of others! Our own competencies, knowledge and skills will help us determine which path we need to follow and what else we need to learn, develop and master in order to get to point B. Even when you face the same fear again and again, just keep on moving.

If you are still not sure which way to go - and trust me, there will be some doubts - prioritize your personal needs and wants. Then align them to your personal and business goals and behaviours that will support those goals. It's really important to know where you are great and where you just suck. So, when you discover what is needed for your business success in terms of your personal goals and interests, begin to think about what resources you should develop, and what you will delegate or outsource.

The thing is – I like to do things differently! Not only because I can, but because I like a dose of risk and excitement. My curiosity is one of my guides. I don't like to work in a boring way. I don't have time for that. The world is changing very quickly. I examine my behaviours to know which actions and reactions I need to change. The very nature of entrepreneurship is that we will go through lots of changes.

What turns you on? What actions do you need to achieve your goal? What else? And what more? Now when you know all of the above, what is your next step? What will you do today?

One day, *Offer Of The Day* appeared on my computer screen - *70% off for 2.500m tandem parachuting*. I knew, it's now or never.

I paid, I agreed, I showed up.

My instructor explained that, if we jump from 2.500m, free fall lasts around 10 seconds, but I can decide to jump from 3.000m or even more, from 3.500m max. What do I get for this investment? The free fall lasts 45 seconds.

I looked at my husband. We were on the same page. In for a penny, in for a pound, as they say in England, I believe. It's once in a blue moon! If this will be so awful, I won't do it again, anyway.

I would be lying if I said I wasn't scared. The seconds passed slowly when we took off by plane and my thoughts were moving at supersonic speed, a speed I couldn't follow. Did I want to quit? Oh yes, many times in a few minutes. But I knew that there would be no second chance.

Be ready for the opportunity. Prepare yourself and hold the line. Set your goal and promise yourself that you will do it. Then do everything that needs to be done.

To make a change, you need the right environment and you need to clear all obstacles and barriers on your path. If you don't like to show up, if you are not self-aware and you overanalyse, you will learn it or burn it. So, when this opportunity comes, you will feel it. Make your decision. Don't overthink it. Just do it!

Ready, steady, jump! Just jump!

Each of us has different experiences, opinions, different values, attitudes and skillsets. We behave differently in different environments. What's working for me doesn't have to work for you.

It's good to have someone who will give you support. Who will encourage you and say: yes, go higher! Who will tap your shoulder when you jump and tell you: *Now spread your arms and fly.* And when you pull the handle of your parachute so hard that you spin in the air and you're sick of it, you'll know – this is part of the learning process.

No one can tell you what you need or must do. If you realize that running your own business isn't for you, that's okay too. Someone at this moment needs you just the way you are. Give your best!

About Renata Ivaštinović

Renata Ivaštinović is a coach for personal and professional development, trainer, business consultant, speaker and author.

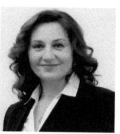

Through workshops, speeches, articles, personal and career development plans, Renata is inspiring teams, entrepreneurs and individuals to take responsibility and achieve beyond their present performance. She is also consulting organizations on how to develop high performing talents. Her coaching programs and trainings are interactive and playful, based on practical business know-how and life's experiences.

Her previous career in leading global companies (L'Oréal, Shell, GlaxoSmithKline etc.) has been developing from operational to managerial roles responsible for establishing and leading Procurement organizations. She led teams through many transitions and transformations and has extensive experience in mentoring and change management coaching.

Renata is a graduate of Silva Mind Control Method - a scientifically proven method of stress control and mind development, is certified Neurolinguistic Coach (NLC), INNLP Practitioner, Wingwave Coach, Wingwave Online Coach and Mindfulness trainer, In-Me.

Contact Renata Ivaštinović

www.renatacoach.com

linkedin.com/in/renata-ivastinovic

Know Your Inner Strength

Simon Fletcher

When I was young, we moved around a lot - Bahrain, Germany, Portsmouth and many other places, before eventually settling in Manchester. My father was a Major in the Army, so I was what they called an army brat. We were never in one place long enough for me to really put down roots or develop a network of friends.

I often felt like I was not good enough, didn't fit in, a bit of a failure. My birth certificate says *Simon Fletcher, Political Agent* because I was born on an army camp in Bahrain where my dad was stationed. It makes me sound special, but I didn't feel very special. I didn't tell kids at school where I was from, I was too embarrassed, and I didn't want to be different. They often tormented me for sounding posh, for not sounding like them. I was ridiculously small for my age and often bullied. I also failed most of my exams because I am dyslexic. It seems to be acceptable to admit you're dyslexic these days but when I was young, you kept it hidden, it was taboo.

At the age of 17, I trained to be a chef. It was exciting, fast-paced and gave me a real buzz.

In those days, Delia Smith and Keith Floyd were the only celebrity chefs. It wasn't trendy like it is these days, no high-profile TV personalities like Gordon Ramsey, Jamie Oliver or Heston Blumenthal. Chef'ing taught me many great, if somewhat critical, life skills, either learn fast or face the wrath of the Head Chef. However, it was a lonely life, not a lot of time for camaraderie in the kitchen, no time for socialising with friends, often working late into the evening and at weekends.

After a few years, I took a massive jump from sweaty kitchens into food sales. It was a massive jump for me because I had to develop new skills, learn technical details about food products, sales targets, and pitching – I had to learn a whole new set of skills, and learning didn't come easy for me! My biggest challenge was trying to get excited and motivated about achieving a 2% increase in sales as opposed to the excitement I felt about the creativity I had been used to as a chef. It was also another lonely job, working by myself, hours, and hours on the road alone in my car. Also, my dyslexia could not be hidden as easily in the sales world, and that felt very vulnerable.

I have had a phenomenally successful sales career. My greatest success was winning a global sales accolade! However, it has always been my dream to give myself a challenge as evidence to prove that I can succeed, that I am not the failure I believed I was. I needed a challenge which would prove that with determination, training and belief in myself – I could do ANYTHING! I want to leave a legacy which would make my son proud of me. I did not want to drift through life, wake up at 93 years old and look back to see that I had not achieved anything.

In 2012, I took on my greatest challenge...

The day came, we sat in the lounge waiting for the word. A year of training in anticipation of THIS day! The phone rang loudly, piercing the eery silence. Garry answers, as we watch in anticipation he slowly turns and smiles, *We're on! Yes!*

We jump with joy, high fives and hugs all round. We run around, grabbing our kit, raiding the fridge, grabbing drinks, whatever we could pack into one small waterproof bag! We climbed aboard the bus and headed off to port. The sun was shining, and skies were blue. I pinched myself to make sure this was not a dream! We felt invincible, like superheroes ready for the challenge!

There she is... our boat for the day... the Captain and the adjudicator are waiting for us. Just so you know how basic this boat is, there was one camping toilet in the bow of the boat, no door, the Captain's cabin was big enough for just the captain and one other person. The only place for us to sit was on boxes on the deck, open to the elements. We climbed aboard, the captain released the ropes, the motor spits out grey blue diesel smoke, chugging away as we set off towards the port gates!

Once out of the port, we circled back towards the shores of Dover.

The first swimmer climbed off the boat and swam back to shore. As she re-entered the cold water, a mere 14-degrees, we all cheered *Come on!* and our Channel Relay Swim began... five swimmers, 21 miles to go (as the crow flies)... note, this did not account for the two metres forward, then one metre back due to the currents!

Then it was my turn to swim.

My heart pumped loud in my chest. I stripped off my warm, dry clothes and felt the sea spray soaking my chest. I stretched, donned my swim cap and goggles and dived in. No wetsuit to protect me. The rules are just speedos!

Looking down into the dark water below, it was so cold, so peaceful. As I set off, salt water on my lips, cold water bashing in my ears, smiling to myself – *This is it, I AM swimming the English Channel!*

For reference, if you are planning to do a solo swim you are only allowed to set off if the weather forecast is gale force 0-1; any higher and you have to wait for better weather. For a relay swim, you can set off if the weather forecast is up to gale force 2. However, as the hours drift by, the weather turns for the worse and the swell getting deeper. As it starts to get dark, we are swimming with flashing white headlights so we could still be seen.

When my turn came to swim again, we were in gale force 7-8. Oddly, it feels safer in the sea!

We pleaded to carry on as the Captain and the adjudicator advised that we needed stop the swim. However, we were only a few miles away from the finish line, we had been swimming for over 12 hours.

Reluctantly, they agree.

I enter the water again and start my next swim, arms and legs powering away. I tucked my head down deep. I need to keep going, I can't let the team down! I feel the power of the sea rocking me. Suddenly, I hear voices screaming and shouting... as I look up, I realise I have been swimming diagonally away from the boat. I stop to get my bearings, then align myself with the boat, head down and start swimming again.

It seems surreal that I feel safer in the sea. As I swim, I disappear deep down into the pit of the swell, dark waves forming high walls around me, the boat disappeared from my view. Next minute, I am riding high on top of the wave, how crazy it seems as now I am peering down at the boat below me!

I finished my session, swim back to the boat, grab the ladders, timing my climb with the swell. On the deck my team-mates cover me with dry towels, as the next person enters the water. I start shivering violently as I try to pull on my clothes, desperate to get warm and desperate for a drink to rinse the sea salt from my mouth. Then I notice the jelly stings all over my legs.

We have done it – 12 hours 52 minutes! We have finished our epic Channel Relay Swim! We wanted to celebrate, but we are in a storm! The Captain said that he would not normally go out above gale force 4, and we were at gale force 8!

The celebration is not what we imagined. We had watched YouTube videos of teams popping champagne, laughing, and dancing in the sun! We celebrated in the dark, in stormy waters, sipping salty champagne exposed to the elements with the waves crashing around us.

It's late, past midnight, as we head back to England. The boat is fighting, crashing against the waves, it feels like we are hitting speed bumps at high speed!

Suddenly, BANG, we hit a big wave and all the lights go out on the boat. I looked desperately at the Captain, his radar and all the digital navigation is dead! SHIT! This can't be happening; I look around expecting to see a film crew shout CUT! We are 15 miles from England, with no lights or navigation, just a small compass to guide us. My inner voice reminds me that we were in one of the busiest waterways in the world. A journey that normally takes an hour took us three, and to add insult to injury, the inflatable boat which was supposed to take us to shore went flat! We pumped it back up, but seawater had flooded the engine, so we had to row back to shore, one person at a time!

What did I learn?

You can achieve anything if your WHY is big enough. And the old adage that you become the people you mix with is so true; team and community are everything. I could not have completed the Channel Relay Swim without the support of my team. And knowing I could not let my team down and they could let me down created a unbreakable bond. And a bond that will never be forgotten…

Oh, and we also raised £2,000 for Cancer Research, BOOM!

Best Life MBA provides a community of like-minded, high achievers who aspire to live to their greatest potential… just like ME… and we all encourage each other to live our Best Life!

About Simon Fletcher

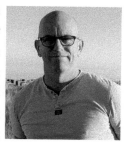

Simon is a highly successful sales professional. He has overcome many personal challenges to achieve global sales accolades. However, Simon's greatest desire was to leave a legacy for his son to be proud of and to prove to himself that he can succeed at any challenge with grit and determination.

Simon faced many challenges in his childhood, as an *army brat* who moved from country to country, he often felt isolated and a bit different from the rest of the school kids. He was also challenged with dyslexia and struggled academically, failing most of his exams.

In 2012, Simon successfully completed his greatest challenge, a Relay Swim across the English Channel in a force 8 gale!

He learned a valuable lesson that he can achieve anything when his WHY is big enough! He has now joined the Best Life MBA community to surround himself with like-minded, high achievers who aspire to live to their greatest potential … just like HIM!

Contact Simon Fletcher

Channel Swim - https://youtu.be/Jv4y4Lpe-ZM

LinkedIn – https://www.linkedin.com/in/simon-fletcher-5651034

Addict to Athlete

Alison Law

For me, leading my best life began when I changed my relationship with alcohol.

My mum was an alcoholic. From the age of 12, I would frequently arrive home from school to find her drunk, then dad would arrive home and they would argue. The arguments would continue through the night. As time went on mum's drinking got worse and the arguments got worse. I would find her drunk in bed in the daytime, incapable of cooking dinner. I learnt not to bring friends home, it was too embarrassing, I didn't want them seeing my mum like that. Sometimes she would make drunken phone calls to my friend's parents crying and I lost friendships. Mum would get drunk, pack her bags and leave, only to be brought home in the early hours of the morning by the police, having found her asleep on someone's front lawn.

Things became unbearable for me and at the age of 15 I took an overdose, ending up in hospital having my stomach pumped. I was discharged with a telling off, that I could have damaged my liver, but no help or support offered.

As I got older, mum and I had terrible rows, I poured her vodka down the sink. She slapped me round the face. We would scream and shout at each other. Mum used to lie about her drinking, dad and I would find loads of empty vodka bottles hidden up the chimney breast and around the house.

After several failed attempts at getting help for her, mum and dad divorced. Mum's drinking escalated. She was jaundiced and had cirrhosis of the liver, her stomach became swollen and she was in pain and was rushed into hospital. They needed to operate; she had an ulcer. I told her I loved her as she was wheeled away, and she told me she loved me, too.

They were the last words she spoke.

She didn't recover from the operation; her body was too weak. Just 24 hours later the nurses quickly called me in, mum's heartbeat was dropping rapidly. Holding my mum's hand, I watched her die. She was only 47.

This had a negative effect on me, at 19, I went down a very dark path. I got involved with the wrong crowds, promiscuity, drugs, and drinking. I found myself in abusive toxic relationships with men with alcohol problems. I went through some horrible times. I cut my wrists on a couple of occasions, not to kill myself but a cry for help. I was taken to hospital but discharged with diazepam with no follow up counselling or support. So, I pretty much got the message that there was no help for me.

I was very much alone, the only way I knew how to get through each day was to self-medicate with alcohol. Twenty plus years passed by of self-medicating and antidepressants and there were so many rock bottoms. When my marriage ended after only six weeks, after I found out he had been cheating. I had a break-down and my drinking became out of control. I was sick, both mentally and physically, I was in a bad place. I realised if I continued, I wouldn't reach 47.

This ignited real change.

I stood in front of the mirror and took an honest look at myself and sobbed. *What had happened to me? Who was I?* I was 44, hungover, fat, unfit, and on anti-depressants. I didn't like what I saw and didn't want to live anymore. I was also a single mum to a beautiful daughter on the Autistic spectrum and she needed me, I had to live. I didn't want her to go through what I had. I decided I was going to change my life.

I wrote a list of what I was gaining from drinking. We never do something without reason, without a why? There must be something to gain otherwise you wouldn't do it.

Mine was to escape and numb the pain I felt.

I realised that everything I thought alcohol had given me, was a lie. It hadn't given me anything but taken them away or made them worse. It contributed to my depression and anxiety. It drained my energy. I lacked motivation, I lost interest in everything. I didn't exercise. I felt ill, sad and lonely. It was the cause of my debt. It took quality time away with my daughter. It stole away my confidence and took away my life.

It was hard to admit, but I was an addict.

So, I poured the remaining alcohol down the sink on New Year's Day, 2017. I filled my fridge with alcohol-free alternatives.

I sought online support and read many self-help books. I joined a gym and a C25K running group.

Gradually, I began to lose weight which helped me make healthier food choices. I set various goals and fitness challenges. Over time, and with consistency my running improved. I entered races and completed my first 5k, 10k, half marathon and eventually a full marathon. I joined a running club and became a Leader in Running Fitness with England Athletics and would lead group runs. I became a Mental Health Ambassador which enabled me to engage with mental health initiatives like run and talk and raise awareness for mental health. I spoke on the local radio about how running had benefited my mental health.

I became interested in self-development and I started really examining my life growing up and what had happened to me.

I found a lady called Lisa A Romano who spoke about co-dependency and narcissistic abuse which all resonated with me.

After further investigation I learnt that my behaviour was due to unresolved childhood trauma. As much as I loved my parents, my mum wasn't emotionally available to me due her alcoholism. Dad had a lot to contend with, so wasn't emotionally available either. There was the fear and shame that my mums drinking brought, the fear of being judged, the anxiety of walking through the door after school, loss of relationships. Not feeling enough, not heard or understood, emotionally neglected, and no one showing me love.

This explained to an extent why I had attracted unhealthy relationships, ones with men who were unavailable in one way or another, who didn't appreciate me, used me, and hurt me. I found myself making excuses for their bad behaviour and believing obvious lies. I put up with the bare minimum of love and attention believing I wasn't worthy of anything else. I was very untrusting and jealous, needy of external validation and never felt safe. I was afraid to set boundaries, in case they left me, I gave them chance after chance hoping things would change. I believed if I did everything I could to please them, did everything they wanted me to do then eventually they would realise how much they loved me and wouldn't leave me.

All I wanted was for someone to love me.

When relationships ended, I was distraught, despite them being dysfunctional. The same feelings as when I lost my mum.

Suddenly it clicked.

When mum died, I had felt abandoned, and here I was feeling abandoned all over again. She chose alcohol over me, which made me think I wasn't a good enough reason for her to live for and if I wasn't good enough for my own mother, how could I be good enough for anyone else. I was seeking the love and validation I never received as a child. The solution was self-love. I had to give the love to myself and stop seeking it from elsewhere.

I am still working on this.

Through this realisation, I had a spiritual experience, I went through great turmoil for several weeks. I didn't know who I was anymore, I didn't feel as though I fitted in, I lost all interest in my usual activities. I lay on the sofa day after day sleeping, crying, and seeking the meaning to my existence.

I read the book *The Power of Now* by Eckhart Tolle and other books on awakening and enlightenment and realised that I was waking up!

I became interested in Buddhism; I wanted a life with no more suffering, and this was the Buddhist path. From here onwards meditation became an important part of my life.

Over the following years, I threw myself into self-improvement, educated myself and completed Diplomas on Alcohol, Drug and Substance Misuse Counselling, and Neuro Linguistic Programming, found voluntary work in addiction recovery groups and became a qualified massage therapist at college part time. I qualified in meditation and mindfulness, too.

I watched a documentary *Awaken The Giant Within* by Tony Robbins and loved it, I began following him on social media.

Through following Tony, I found Jean-Pierre De Villiers. I read about his accident and then followed him with admiration on his miraculous journey of recovery, his strength and determination to recover was astounding and utterly inspirational. I read *How To Own Your Life* and it inspired me so much, it gave me the motivation to continue my journey. Understanding how taking responsibility and owning where I was in my life was a game changer for me.

When I saw JP had a coaching community, I was so excited, I signed up immediately, and I'm now part of *Best Life MBA*, the coaching and support is amazing, it's one of the best decisions I've ever made.

This year I really challenged myself mentally and physically.

In May, I ran my marathon virtually. In June, I ran 100 mile in seven days. In July, I took on an epic challenge of virtually running the distance from Land's End to John O'Groats, 874 miles in 12 weeks. This was huge for me, but I believed I could do it. I knew it was all about mindset, like the quote by Henry Ford says, *Whether you think you can or you can't, you're right.*

I did have moments of doubt.

It was tough getting up and running every day, sometimes twice, regardless of tiredness or weather. I kept thinking of what I've been through in my life and that this wasn't anywhere near as tough as the pain I had already endured, and that kept me going. Not only did I complete it, but I completed it three weeks earlier and finishing it with another marathon. Then, three weeks later I ran my third marathon The Virtual London Marathon and achieved a PB.

I think it might be OK to say now that I am an athlete!

I'm 47 now, and I'm the fittest, healthiest, and happiest I've ever been. I would never have been able to achieve any of these things had I not stopped drinking. There have been a couple of slip ups along the way, but no one's perfect and it's nothing to be ashamed of, its all part of the journey.

Addiction is about so much more, it's about mental health, self-awareness, self-belief, and confidence that you can change your life, reinvent yourself, if you really want to.

I don't blame my mum or anyone else. I love her so much and miss her every day. I'm sure she would be extremely proud of me. I take full responsibility for everything that's happened to me. I'm thankful for the experiences and what they've taught me. I now want to use these to help others. Every day is another opportunity to turn your life around. I'm a new person, I've got a new life, a better life, in fact, I'm now living my best life.

About Alison Law

Alison Law is a single mum to a daughter on the Autistic Spectrum. She has worked in various voluntary settings from supporting adults with additional needs to mentoring in support groups for substance misuse. She was voted *Volunteer Of The Year 2016*.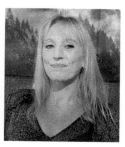

Alison is a published Author and Poet.

As well as a qualified Massage Therapist, she has Diploma's in Counselling, Alcohol, Drug and Substance Misuse Counselling, Neuro Linguistic Programming, Meditation and Mindfulness.

She is an Ultra-Running athlete, a qualified Leader in Running Fitness for England Athletics, and a Mental Health Ambassador. Her passions lie in helping people in their recovery from addiction, mental health, and self -improvement.

Her mission is to encourage talking about addiction and mental health to promote awareness and reduce the stigma surrounding it and to inspire others to transform their lives

Contact Alison Law

Instagram: @sobergirl72

Facebook: Sober Minds

Website: www.soberminds.co.uk

When You Change, Everything Changes

Brady George

It wasn't so long ago that my life was very different from the way it is today. I got started in business young, discovered I was good at it and put it above everything else in my life. It was the fuel that powered my existence. Consequently, by the time I celebrated my 27th birthday, I was the archetypal ambitious business leader; a fully paid-up subscriber to the classic notion that *work hard, play hard* was the *only* route to success.

Unfortunately, like so many who adopted that same strategy before me, I found that working hard and playing hard became an addiction that I found I couldn't control any more. I was becoming drunk on work, consuming it as intently and consistently as an alcoholic might down shots at a bar. I don't doubt those around me noticed my intoxication with a growing sense of alarm, but for a long time, I didn't see the problem.

I was chasing the business dream and doing pretty well, I thought.

No matter that my physical health was taking a hit in the meantime: overweight, unfit, unhealthy and, ultimately, feeling tired continually and drained. That's just the price you pay for success, right? *Go hard or go home*, I'd tell myself.

From the outside peering in, I must have looked a mess.

Snatching fragments of sleep that probably totalled maybe three or four hours a night, my routine was lousy.

The weight continued to pile on, but for some reason, I hadn't yet made the connection between the gradual destruction of my body and the lifestyle I was leading. You know those TV shows where they get doctors and specialists to assess a person's health and, at the end of the show, tell them what their body age is? I would have been a prime candidate for those programmes, and the findings would have been ugly. Perhaps they'd have told me my body was twice as *old* as I actually was? Maybe even worse.

Aside from the physical damage I was causing myself, eventually, the mental damage started taking its toll, too.

I was in a constant state of fight or flight and suffering with acute stress. Pains in my chest and arms became the norm and car journeys became the place to scream, shout and cry. Small wonder, given my attitude to life.

That attitude was, of course, something that had been cultivated within me as I grew up. I'd been working with my father for four years or so by this point, and he's a man who has always demonstrated a strong work ethic. I watched him, learned from him and, like most developing boys and young men, in many respects, I copied him too. Or at least I thought that's what I was doing – in reality, my father was simply instilling the value of hard work in me, not encouraging me to take it to this extreme. He certainly wasn't telling me to stop taking care of myself.

By this point, I considered everything that didn't fit into *work hard, play hard* an unnecessary distraction. Hobbies, leisure time, keeping fit, relationships and so on were all just pointless complications that other people wasted energy on. I didn't have time for anything so profligate.

Then, inevitably, my world came crashing down.

My lifestyle drove me to a serious health scare and forced me to a complete stop. Being confined to my bed for two weeks, utterly exhausted, was not something that fitted in with my approach to life. I had so much I should have been doing, and every second I stayed in bed, the clock next to me ticked away as if it was taunting my inactivity. The lost hours felt like a failure, when in fact, as I realise now, they were a huge victory.

Because being trapped in that bed for a fortnight was my escape out of the spiral I'd become locked in. It gave me time to think, to reflect on what I was doing to myself, and to wake up. This was the moment when I realised something was fundamentally wrong and had to change. It was the moment when I decided that I had to take better care of my health. I had to start getting fit.

I should say at this point that I didn't mean I was suddenly going to quit my directorial job and something else. I just enjoyed leading a business and had no plans to give everything up. But I realised there was a better, more rounded way to be successful, and that started with finding somewhere to train that would fit in around the work commitments I wanted to keep.

So, I started looking and asking around for a personal trainer who would be prepared to help me kick myself into shape either very early in the morning or very late in the evening. And one day, I found Jules Taylor. Jules is a legend of a man. An endurance coach, a triple Ironman, a guy who has practically done it all in the sporting world. He also seemed, well, a tiny bit crazy. In a good way, if you know what I mean. Not only did he agree to train me before five in the morning, he actively encouraged it. Jules is a rare breed.

Naturally, I checked out his bio online before we met. To say it made me somewhat daunted and apprehensive before our first session would be a massive understatement. There I was, heavily overweight and in the worst shape of my life, getting out of my car to meet a guy who was essentially my life opposite in that regard. I'd get out of breath climbing a flight of stairs. Jules is the sort of guy who'd consider an epic run to the top of the Shard *lap one*.

On that first, pre-dawn morning in April with Jules, I took a 45-minute fitness test. The initial ten seconds were fine. After that, I didn't fare well. By 5:45am, the test was at an end and so, effectively, was I. Curled up in a ball on the changing room floor, I focused all my remaining energy on the challenge of trying to keep hold of my breakfast. I was dizzy, entirely spaced out, and the room was spinning like a fairground waltzer. If a human body is supposed to be made up of 60% water, then it felt as if the whole lot had leeched out of my skin, turned to sweat and started evaporating into the chilly morning air. It was all I could do to gather myself sufficiently to stumble out of the gym changing room and mutter, "Thanks," to Jules before I left. Only a few months earlier, it would have been impossible for me to imagine thanking another human being for providing me with this experience!

As I slumped into my car seat and wearily pulled the door closed behind me, I realised I needed to make a long-overdue commitment to my physical health. I needed to envision a more self-supporting future for myself and prioritise something that I had neglected for far too long. I didn't know it at the time, but this was my first taste of non-negotiability.

The weeks, even the months, that followed were tough but incredibly rewarding. I made a non-negotiable promise to myself to change an aspect of my life around, and that vow created a good habit which, in turn, created more good habits.

Within the space of 12 months, I dropped 25 pounds – over 11 kilos – in weight. I was happier, healthier and more productive. Who doesn't want to say that about their life?

I began transitioning towards a more plant-based diet and even started swapping my old, unhealthy food and drink routine for revitalising bright green detox juices. It was one positive switch after another. But I never gave up on that 5am appointment with myself. All this change was only able to take place because I decided to make a non-negotiable commitment to train for the benefit of my health. To follow through with it and to never quit no matter what. It seems like such a simple little act, in a way, but the power it has is truly unbelievable.

It doesn't matter how many New Year's Resolutions you make – to give up smoking, to eat less chocolate, to save money in a pension – if you don't make them non-negotiable, your chances of success reduce drastically. You need to front up to yourself and know that there's no way out of following through on what you've set out to achieve. Sure, you're going to fall off the wagon occasionally – hands up, it happens to me too – but if that's the case, don't beat yourself up about it because it doesn't make anything better. Just dust yourself down and climb straight back on. Even with small hiccups along the way, the intense strength of your non-negotiable promise will guide you to your ultimate goal.

Who knows what bonuses you'll encounter along the way too? For me, it was meeting up with some of Jules' other clients: highly successful businesspeople who became part of my network and opened up a whole new world of possibilities that I, as a *twentysomething* business owner, had never known were available.

That 5am April battering I took from Jules' fitness test has served me well in so many ways.

I met JP De Villiers 8 years ago in Tenerife at a Tony Robbins' seminar and 18 months ago got back in touch for some private coaching.

Since then, I haven't stopped making non-negotiable commitments, and I haven't stopped taking my personal fitness seriously, either.

In 2020, for instance, I finished my first Ironman triathlon and completed the 4/4/48 challenge – a demanding physical endeavour popularised by ex-Navy Seal fitness guru, David Goggins, involving running four miles every four hours for 48 hours. I wonder what my 27-year-old self would say if he could see me now?

He certainly wouldn't recognise my new mantra. No longer

governed by the false idol of *work hard, play hard*, the critical principle in my life now is: *when you change, everything changes*.

I live my life with that phrase permanently etched into my mind. Although that sometimes means having to be brave and more courageous to achieve it, to do so creates possibilities that you didn't realise were even there or that you were capable of. There's an associated quote from Dr Brené Brown that always really resonates with me: *You can choose courage, or you can choose comfort, but you cannot choose both.*

Think about that for a second.

I have to be honest and admit that I undoubtedly received incredible support from those around me along the way. My fiancé, Taya, stood by me through the rough times when I must have been nigh-on permanently absent as a partner. She has always been my rock. And now that I'm fortunate enough to be a father to two gorgeous daughters, the ability to be non-negotiable with myself is more crucial than ever. I must be there for them as a proper father, and I must demonstrate to them through my own actions that looking after yourself is an enormously important part of being human.

The moment that you choose to harness the power of being non-negotiable, your life changes. Suddenly, you understand that you aren't on the journey, you are the journey. Your life's meaning and message to the world are manifestations of who you become.

When you change, everything changes. What are you going to change? Who are you becoming?

About Brady George

Brady is an international, multiple award winning, property and outsourced services expert, entrepreneur, vegan athlete and CEO of the Almeda Group a facilities management provider serving a client market cap of over $120Bn.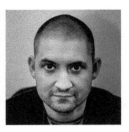

A life partner to Taya and a very proud father to his two daughters Isla and Harper, Brady is dedicated to living his very best life.

In 2016, Brady was awarded the prestigious award as the UK director of the year by the *Institute Of Directors* (IOD) for his contribution and vision for corporate social responsibility. He is regularly asked to speak on business and industry led topics. Brady trained at the Cranfield School of Management.

Contact Brady George

www.almedagroup.com

https://www.linkedin.com/in/bradygeorge/

https://www.instagram.com/bradyggeorge/

Living The Dream

Angela Fletcher

"I have a dream" - Martin Luther King

Like many, I have a dream, and I'd like to take you on my rollercoaster ride so far.

Imagine, a sunny afternoon in the mid 1960's, my sister and I were happily throwing grass into a river and giggling as it disappeared along the bubbling current. I heard a splash and as I turned, the image of my little sister, face down in the river burned into my memory forever. Months later, as I sat playing with my dolls on the lounge floor, I quietly said, "Mummy, can you ask Baby Jesus to bring Carrie home now, I miss her."

I often felt sad and lonely as I was growing up, and different somehow. So, my dream became a simple one: *When I grow up, I want to get married, have two children and a happy family.*

And be ordinary.

When I was 23, I was happily married and pregnant with our first child. On 23rd March 1988, I gave birth to a beautiful baby boy, Jamie. We were living the dream! But Jamie died shortly after he was born due to birth complications. I remember feeling like was my fault, I must have done something terribly wrong during my pregnancy.

I carried the same fear and guilt throughout my second pregnancy a year later, fearing the same fate for our second son, Lewis. Perhaps we were too young and naïve to know how to handle our grief, but our marriage didn't survive the loss of Jamie and we eventually divorced.

My hopes and dreams for a happy family were crushed.

At 26, I met my soulmate, Jay who asked me to marry him just three short weeks after we met, and I excitedly said "Yes". 18 months later, we married beneath the blazing sun on the golden sands of Antigua, with Lewis as our proud best man. We were living the dream! But 12 months later, just three days before our first wedding anniversary, Jay lost his short battle with cancer. As his life slipped away from him, my hopes and dreams slipped away from me, and grief consumed me once more.

I was still recovering from my grief when I met Simon.

Simon showed me how to laugh again, my knight in shining armour, come to take me across the bridge to happiness. His proposal was a grand romantic gesture, he surprised me with choosing the perfect wedding venue and he found our perfect dream home. We got married, we had our perfect little boy, Harrison, we were living the dream! But, as the years rolled by, we let life get in the way, we were no longer the happy family that I had always dreamed of, we were no longer living the dream.

One day, after a huge fight, we split up. But, after a short separation, we agreed that we wanted to make our marriage work and keep our family together. We took a short, romantic break to rekindle our passion, restore our love for each other and hopefully rescue our marriage!

We sat in a hot tub in the depths of the forest, sipping champagne and giggling like a couple of newlyweds, stars sparkling like diamonds in the night sky above us!

However, I had a knot in the pit of my stomach, a niggling doubt that I couldn't shake off ...

We had some big issues to deal with!

Once again, I was consumed by grief at the possible loss of my marriage, but I gradually realised that this time I had a choice – should I stay, or should I go? It was the hardest decision I've ever had to make but I chose to stay.

If you have read JP's story, you will know that following his hit-and-run cycling accident he set himself a stretch goal for his recovery, to summit Mount Kilimanjaro. Now, Simon and I stood at the foot of our own mountain, a mountain of recovery to re-discover who we really are, a journey back to us, individually and as a couple.

My quest began immediately, my search for meaning in this mess.

First step... we found ourselves a brilliant therapist. Next step and the next and the next... we read book after book after book. We started healing the marriage wound, restoring trust, healing our inner child. We started developing our understanding and capacity for self-care, compassion, empathy, vulnerability, courage, love, relationships, happiness and much, much more. Our immediate focus was to get the help *we needed.*

About a year into our soul-searching journey, whilst at a Tony Robbins seminar, digging deep and uncovering our limiting beliefs... I came to a sudden, stark, shocking realisation – we both brought a lot of baggage into our relationship.

Slowly, I began to realise that I had clung onto past traumas as my story, unprocessed memories from my childhood which had probably shaped my view that the world was an unsafe place. Loss after loss, which had probably wired my perception and cultivated my limiting beliefs that *nobody will stay with me, I don't deserve love, I don't deserve to be happy.* I had brought all my doubts and fears into our marriage and had never realised how much they kept me from living my best life, bringing my best self into relationships, including my marriage.

I had been getting in my own way the whole of my life and never even realised it!

Today, I have a new dream!

My dream is to leave my career of 35 years in the corporate world and become a full-time Relational Trauma Coach, a published author and an international speaker. My dream is to give hope and courage to others and their families, who find themselves standing at the foot of that same mountain that Simon and I stood before, wondering whether they will ever be able to make the long climb to the top and beyond. My dream is to be a beacon of hope that marriages can survive relational wounds and rise from the ashes to become much more intimate and fulfilling relationships than they have ever been.

I completed the training to become a life coach, I completed the training to become a relational trauma coach, I continued to read hundreds of books and attended every webinar and event that I could find relating to self-development, healing trauma, recovering from whatever life throws at you, healing your past!! I joined a Facebook community and supported hundreds of partners walking the healing path with me. However, I still clung onto my corporate job, scared of letting go of the certainty it gave me, scared of taking the leap into that scary, unsafe world. I was still full of fear and uncertainty – *I can't start my own business, I'm not good enough to earn a living as a coach.* Oh, those limiting beliefs and critical self-talk – my absolute best friends! I realised I needed to do much, much more work on loving and believing in myself.

I love Adam Roa's wonderful poem, *You Are Who You Have Been Looking For*, which was inspired when he learned your capacity to love others is limited only by your capacity to love yourself. In his poem he asks, *If you can't love yourself, how could you ever love me?* and urges us to *treat yourself like someone you love.* So …

… how do you live *Your Best Life?*

Love yourself first! Prioritise yourself above all others… identify your limiting beliefs and then chuck them out with the bath water – *You Are Already Enough* (Adam Roa).

I have now left the corporate world! I AM starting my own business as a Relational Trauma Coach. I AM writing a book (starting with this chapter) and I AM speaking on public stages. I am the only authentic ME there is in this world and my life's purpose is to serve others who have been crushed by life, particularly in their marriage, to show them hope and give them courage to heal their wounds!

About Angela Fletcher

Angela is a successful Relational Trauma coach, public speaker and published author.

Her journey as coach began in 2017 when her marriage threatened to be torn apart by traumas past and present.

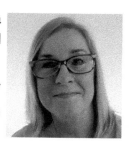

She and her husband faced the long road of recovery together as they each fought to overcome and heal the emotional wounds of their traumas to save their marriage.

Angela left the security of her corporate job to devote herself to becoming a beacon of hope for others in the same situation. Her mission is to be a beacon of hope that marriages can survive relational wounds and rise from the ashes to become a much more intimate and fulfilling relationship than it has ever been.

Angela has successfully coached and mentored 100's of betrayed partners through individual coaching and group support in a Facebook community. She has developed a relationship and recovery coaching programme to provide couples with the information and tools they need to heal their own trauma and restore their relationships.

Contact Angela Fletcher

www.angela-fletcher.co.uk

https://linktree/angela.fletcher

Everything Happens On The Last Attempt

Francisco Bricio

I have been fortunate to be good at maths since I remember. I was one of the smart kids at school: straight As, an avid reader, and I love classical music, Mahler, in particular. I'm a physicist who is very good with computers.

My first serious job was for a 2,000-employee software company in Houston. Apparently, I was the only person who passed the maths and statistics tests that a large round of applicants went through, so they offered me a job on the spot even though I barely spoke English at that time.

In ten years, I rapidly grew from a clerical position on the lower ranks to become Vice President of Sales for Latin America, with a six-figure salary flying in the corporate jet.

The company rewarded creativity generously, so I designed an algorithm to find massive financial opportunities hidden under layers and layers of corporate data from different software platforms in my free time.

When I finished, I presented it to Bob, the company president; he loved the algorithm's design, simplicity and elegance. He invited me for dinner the next day at his beautiful mansion in the suburbs.

I must say that I didn't expect this; after all, Bob was a very private person, and only a handful of his very close allies had been to his house for dinner.

So, I created this idea in my mind that I was going to be rewarded with a huge bonus; instead, he asked me to leave the company and use my project to start a new business on my own.

I was devastated.

He insisted that I was *ready* to become an entrepreneur; that I had learnt everything I needed to know. I told him I didn't have the enormous resources a company like that required.

He asked me to calculate how much money I needed and asked me to work on a business plan and a one-page summary and meet him again the following Monday.

I remember sitting in my dining room late on Sunday night with my head fixed at the numbers on the page. The numbers were perfect, but my heart didn't want to leave the company.

In a desperate attempt to stay, almost by survival instinct, I crossed out all the numbers, multiplied every amount by three, printed the final copy, and went to bed.

The next morning, Bob was already waiting for me, sharp on time.

I've had many *What does this mean?* and *Why am I here?* moments in my life - and this was the first one of many.

Are you ready?

Yes, I said, as I passed him a folder with the one-page summary he asked for.

He took the piece of paper, quickly glanced, looked at the big number at the bottom, put the page down, and asked me:

When do you want to start?

I was shocked! I didn't know what to say!

Oh! Hold on Bob, what about the money? Is this going to be a loan with interest? What's the interest rate?

No, it is <u>not</u> a loan.

So, are we going to be partners? What percentage of the company do you want in exchange?

No, we are <u>not</u> going to be partners.

Sorry Bob, I don't understand…

He looked straight to me and solemnly uttered only two words: *Pay Forward.*

I didn't respond, so he continued. "Many years ago, someone did with me the same thing I'm doing with you. The money you asked for is yours under three conditions:

1. You need to put blood, sweat, and tears to make this the best product on the market. Where everyone else has given up, you will find additional strength to continue.

2. We will meet every five years. You will tell me about your progress,

and I'll be ruthless on my critique and expectations. I will not accept any excuses.

3. Pay Forward. You need to start looking for someone with potential, and when ready, you need to help that person start his own business with whatever amount asked. And even if that person comes to you with a number three times larger than necessary, you need to say yes right away..."

I was so embarrassed and was going to apologize for my desperate attempt to increase the numbers so he would say no. But he raised his hand in to express that he knew precisely how much this project would cost and that there was nothing for me to apologize for.

Next week I was back in Mexico, wealthy and working on the product, and one year later, we were ready to sell.

The product's success resided in having companies anonymously share their accounting information with other companies so that everyone would benefit from comparable benchmarks; something very attractive to every company I talked to, but no one wanted to be the first one to share their data.

Days became weeks, weeks became months, and months became years of expenses with no income. Everyone liked the product, but no one wanted to be the first one to buy.

By the end of the fourth year, I had not only drained the original money Bob gave me, but I was already under terrible financial pressure caused by a series of loans that I had acquired to continue operating the company.

I owed millions, MILLIONS.

Things turned ugly very rapidly, lawyers, collectors, phone threats, embargo, eviction, and we didn't have enough money to eat. We were starving.

We couldn't continue living like this. It was not fair for my wife and our three daughters. After reviewing the terms of my life insurance, I made up my mind. I was worth more dead than alive. My family was going to be in a better position if I was not around.

My wife found me crying in the bathroom. She asked me to calm down, asked me to call Bob, and, like the parable of the prodigal son in the Bible, to tell him the truth: That I had lost everything he gave me and to ask him to take me back as *as one of your hired servants.*

The next morning, with my wife beside me, I called him. He was not there yet, so I left him a message that I would call him back later.

As soon as I hung up, the phone rang again. It was a call from one of the largest corporations in the country, the man on the other side of the line sounded foreign. He told me that he had just arrived in the country, that he was the new director, and that he has been briefed that I had a product that he had been looking for many years. He asked me to make a presentation the next day in Mexico City.

If this had been in another time, I would have jumped on the first plane to see him. But at that point, I had no money. I couldn't afford to buy a ticket to Mexico City, which is 600 kilometers from where I live.

So, in an attempt to save face, I politely said, "Thanks, but no thanks. I have been in your company numerous times, and

I know you like the product, but you never make up your mind, and I can't waste any more time with you."

He responded: "If you come tomorrow and what I see is what I've been told you have, you will have a purchase order. I promise".

I don't know why I said I would be there. But as soon as I hung up, I looked at my wife with the look of someone in trouble: *I didn't have the money for the trip.*

A few hours later, my wife came with a small handful of dollar bills. She had sold the small antique coin I gave her at our wedding at the pawnshop.

The money was barely enough for a round bus trip, nothing else, so I couldn't even pay for a hotel.

I took the night bus to arrive in Mexico City early in the morning, clean myself at the bus station bathroom, be on time for the meeting and take the bus back home.

It was a one-shot deal. And I got it!

Today, my company has more than 2,000 clients in 11 countries.

I am an advisor to two of the largest car manufacturers in the world and a member of several companies' board of directors.

I also participate in three other businesses - biomedical, insurance and high-tech industries - and I am an investor in several more.

Besides my three beautiful daughters, my wife and I support

two more girls who had penurious childhoods. And we also support the foster house where they came from.

I'm the president of Sociedad Mahler; one of the society's activities is a music conservatory for more than two hundred under-privileged children in Irapuato, Mexico. We want them to learn music instead of being on the streets.

I'm also the Vice-Chairman of the Mahler Foundation. This worldwide non-profit organization promotes and carries the legacy of the music of Gustav Mahler around the world.

Life has been good to me. I feel blessed and I will live my life in eternal gratitude.

Everything happens on the last try; nothing happens on the first, second, or any numbered try.

So stop counting. Things always happen on the very last attempt.

Never give up. You never know if your breakthrough lies behind the attempt you are thinking of giving up.

About Francisco Bricio

Francisco Bricio is a theoretical physicists, technology and automotive retail expert,

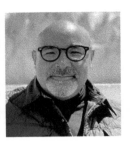

He is the founder of Simetrical, Vice-Chairman of The Mahler Foundation and President of the Sociedad Mahler.

He lives in Guadalajara Mexico with his wife and daughters.

Contact Francisco Bricio

Web Address: https://franciscobricio.com

LinkedIn: https://www.linkedin.com/in/franciscobricio/

Instagram: https://www.instagram.com/franciscobricio/

Twitter: https://twitter.com/franciscobricio

Perception! Perception! Perception!

Yvette L Baker

When my mother was receiving end-of-life care, I kept vigil by her bedside day and night. It was an honour and a privilege to be there. It could have been a wretched, cheerless time but I knew that mum's suffering would soon be over. I chatted to mum as though she could hear and understand all that I was saying.

Every other day my siblings visited and we'd laugh and share memories of our childhood. Never did I feel maudlin or anguished. My mum looked beautiful. I washed her face, I bathed her lips, brushed her hair, held her hand and kissed her. I had a playlist of her favourite songs which filled the room with joy.

Her last night felt like the end of an incredible holiday. The October sunset over the adjacent parkland was beautiful and I described it to my mum, pretending that we were on some exotic island, packed and ready to leave next morning. I stayed awake all that night, listening to my mum's breath slowly changing. At 10.02am she breathed her last. Finally, she'd checked out. I smiled knowing that my playlist must have been truly awesome!

Life – ephemeral, fleeting, short-lived and temporary. We live, we die. We all know it, but the idea can be a stark, brutal and worrying notion.

So how do we cope knowing that we have an end date, and that built-in obsolescence is a reality? I'm reminded of a rhyme my children used to chant with hand actions - *Here is Buggy, Buggy say hi, Buggy fly high, Buggy fly low, Buggy die.* Between *Buggy fly low and Buggy die* was a dramatic pause as poor little Buggy hit a window and perished. Poor Buggy. A quick lesson in the impermanence of life.

Buggy's demise reminds me of a whimsical ditty my grandmother used to sing: *Doctor, Doctor will I die? Yes, my dear and so shall I.* A short refrain, addressing death succinctly and perfectly.

I grew up with the understanding that our time on earth is finite and that one day we will no longer be here, so the concept has never scared or worried me. It's just one of those things that will happen one day and I'm sanguine about that. My grandmother, wittingly I'm sure, set me up for all the deaths and near misses that were to follow and are still to come, including my own which I choose to face with calm equanimity.

I was born in 1965 to my mother a nurse and my father a linguist. I had two siblings – a sister and younger brother. My brother was born with cerebral palsy, infantile fits and cognitive disabilities so categorised as educationally subnormal (ESN). This must have been a devastating blow to my parents who, despite everyone's advice to put my brother in a home and leave him there, decided to keep him with them and us. Although this meant that we had a baby brother, this put a considerable strain upon my parents' mental health and marriage.

My brother screamed for weeks and weeks when he first came home – a high-pitched scream and cry which was disturbing for all. The GP dismissed my mother as neurotic and said that this was normal behaviour for a baby. Of course, it wasn't and my mum knew that instinctively. It turned out that, on top of everything else, he had a hiatus hernia which after many months was corrected. This knocked my mum's confidence and depression took hold. Mother's Little Helper - Valium was prescribed, and the smiling, gentle mummy of my early years, was replaced by a short-tempered, withdrawn, emotionally distant, skinny, gaunt, disinterested lady, who graduated to Prozac and various other fashionable anti-depressants. When I was around 20 she confessed that she couldn't remember my sister and I as children. That was one of the saddest and most poignant moments of my life, and perhaps hers too.

Mum seemed to spend a lot of time staring into the distance, lost in thought and smoking. (A habit she'd picked up as a cadet nurse).

As a child, I wanted to reach out and protect her, so gave her lots of love and cuddles. She in turn would stroke my inner arm in a very soothing way. I would nestle up to her on the sofa enjoying the warmth and scent of her body. The security of those cuddles was powerful. Even though emotionally she was distant and unreachable, she was my mum and I loved her unconditionally.

Always knowing that my mum, despite her sadness and depression, was in there kept me going. I put a smile on my face and refused to be miserable. I was the family clown. The joker. I probably suppressed a lot, but the smiles and the laughter became part of me. I also enjoyed quiet time and alone time. I've never been one for loud parties and big groups, but I do love the companionship of people and I love listening to their stories. Being quiet and having serenity were qualities of my grandmother and I regarded them highly.

One spring morning, when I was about five years old, and getting ready for school, an old lady knocked on our front door. She had found a little girl wandering around outside our house crying. It was the daughter of our next-door neighbour and my best friend, Anita. My mum invited Anita in, thanked the lady and instructed us to wait inside and said she'd return shortly. Of course, being a curious child, I wanted to know what was happening, so I rather pompously instructed Anita to wait for me and slipped out of the front door to follow my mum.

Although I was just moments behind her, she didn't realise and we both entered the house. The sight in front of us was shocking. Slumped against the sofa in the middle of the lounge was Anita's mum, Mags. Blue in colour, unresponsive and to the untrained eyes of a 5-year-old, looking very dead indeed.

It was actually quite fascinating to see a body in such a condition. A lady who I really liked and now seemingly gone. I wanted to touch her, but my mum shook her head. I could not turn my eyes away from this almost-corpse. I was riveted. I wanted to know why she'd turned blue. Why she wasn't her normal colour. Why she was unable to speak. Why she was staring like that. As my mum dialled for an ambulance, she pointed to a bottle of pills at Mags' side, which seemed to offer an answer. Mags was whisked away to hospital and for weeks after adults spoke in hushed tones. Fortunately, she survived. I found out later that she was in a desperately sad and loveless marriage, with four children and felt so trapped that suicide seemed to be her only choice.

Over the years, deaths followed: family, friends, friends' children and acquaintances. Some sudden and unexpected, others less so. Death often arouses powerful emotions, but the ritual of death and the realisation that we are here but temporarily is liberating and completely takes the sting out of it for me.

My mum had dementia, diverticulitis, COPD and lung cancer. However, it was a fall that precipitated her death. I mention her ill-health, because in my role as a holistic therapist, I work with the principles of Traditional Chinese Medicine. Five interdependent elements - Fire, Earth, Metal, Water and Wood which support and control one another but when out of balance sanction dis-ease.

The element of Metal corresponds to the lungs and the large intestine. The emotion associated with metal is grief and sadness. Interestingly, my mum experienced a lot of trauma, sadness and grief in her lifetime. My mum internalised and suppressed her suffering and so the dis-ease that she felt, in time grew so great and became so unbearable that it led to disease.

I believe that you can positively influence your health by just altering your perception and using positivity to nourish body, mind and soul. Healthy diet, exercise, breathing, thinking happy thoughts and finding the good even in stressful situations leads to resilience. Rather than transmitting anger, sadness, pessimism and negativity to the 40 trillion or so cells in your body, try smiling, laughing and meditating.

Clients often come to me as a last resort, when their symptoms are causing them great distress. The integrity of the immune system is compromised with repeated stress and the body less able to fight infection. Pathogens multiply and tissues degrade. By changing the way we think about our stressors, the ability to cope with them is increased and we become less susceptible to stress related diseases.

I see modern disease daily: high blood pressure, heart attack, migraine, IBS, diabetes, anxiety, depression, infertility and more. Micro stresses have built up and worries, fears and anxieties are internalised. Clients describe themselves as just going through the motions. Through discussion, reflexology, massage, Reiki or meditation, relief occurs and the body's self-healing process is activated and wellbeing improved.

In a world which has the potential to be gloomy and sad we have two choices – to view it through a lens of fear and anxiety or one of cheerful positivity. Like a kaleidoscope and its ever-changing patterns – some combinations are harmonious, others discordant. With a quick twist the view is changed forever. Our lives are rich and full and we have to experience all colours to appreciate the differences and to learn from them. By eliminating our own anger, fear and resentment the world will be seen in all its glory and we'll no longer be afraid. Cultivating warmth, compassion, integrity and love and being kind to others regardless of what they say, do or think, brings goodness, light and freedom to our lives. That is magical and will help you sparkle. It will lift you and make you feel bright, effervescent and free. Remember, it's all about perception.

About Yvette L Baker

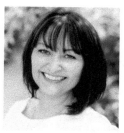

Holistic therapist and published author Yvette, teaches meditation, runs retreats, wellbeing sessions, mentors trainee reflexology and massage therapists, all delivered in person and online.

She is passionate about the positive effects that reflexology, massage, meditation and Reiki can have on the physical, mental and emotional aspects of the body. Yvette knows that by treating you as a whole, your spirit for life will be lifted and balance, harmony and calm restored.

Yvette consistently enables her clients to attain optimum health. She knows that health is not a luxury, but a right and that we can all be proactive about this. By encouraging and supporting her clients through their challenges, she helps them to discover the right path. Conditions she has treated include, motor neurone disease, Parkinson's, Alzheimers, diabetes, fibromyalgia, MS, cancer, lymphoedema, depression, infertility and many more.

Her favourite karaoke song is *On Top of the World* by the Carpenters!

Contact Yvette L Baker ITEC MAR MFHT

https://www.harmonyholisticscalne.co.uk

Facebook: https://www.facebook.com/harmonyholisticscalne

https://www.instagram.com/harmony_holistics_calne

Your Failures Do Not Define You

Gavin J Gallagher

Back in July 2008 I had it all. There is a particular moment that I remember like it was yesterday - it was a beautiful sunny morning and I was with my 4-year old daughter Amber in the South of Spain. We had just woken up in our new 5-bedroom villa and the first thing she wanted to do was jump in our new swimming pool. I remember pinching myself as we played in the water thinking to myself, *"Yep, I could get used to this."*

My wife was back in Dublin with our other two daughters, 2-year old Ashley and new-born Alicia. We had decided to pack up our beautiful Dublin home and relocate to Spain for a few years so I could pursue an ambitious new real estate project that I started the year before. I had been very active back in Ireland, but this new Spanish project was the one, and I was convinced it was going to change everything.

The previous five years had been the most active in my life – half a decade buying and selling real estate, doing deals, developing buildings and renting them to tenants. They called this period the *Celtic Tiger* and as a successful 35-year old,

I considered myself one of the new tiger cubs. It was a time when, if you were hungry you could make a lot of money very quickly, provided you didn't mind taking risks. Big risks meant big rewards so I went all-in.

I was not a big property name by any stretch of the imagination, but I was doing very well, luck seemed to favour me and my lucky streak had been running now for five years straight. Everything I touched seemed to turn to gold - one property I bought quadrupled in value, I sold another for a €2.5 million profit just 6-weeks after buying it.

I was on a rocket ship.

During this time banks were falling over themselves to lend me money - one offered me a special credit card with a dedicated concierge service and a €40,000 a month credit limit. Did I need it? No. Did I take it? Of course I did! Every time I borrowed money I would just make more, so it didn't take long to get addicted. A self-described debt junkie I even started borrowing to invest in the stock market, quickly turning €100,000 into €850,000 in less than six months.

The problem with rapid success is it goes straight to the head – your ego can be a dangerous thing. I got sloppy and complacent, paying less attention to detail and more to having a good time. I had the flashy car, the big house, the holiday villa and a love for all things luxury and first class. The worst thing about a lucky streak is that the longer it runs the more convinced you become that you are invincible, that you can do no wrong.

Fast forward three years and the world was a different place – the Global Financial Crisis had happened and those same banks that couldn't lend me money fast enough were now calling me constantly, demanding it all back. The big project that was going to change everything was sitting empty and the investors were calling me up looking for updates on how it was doing.

How on earth did I end up here?

My beautiful 7-bedroom mansion in Dublin was gone, sold at a 70% discount to what it had been worth in 2008. My investments were all valued well below what I had paid for them, even my stock market portfolio had reversed leaving me with a €250,000 hole to fill, but hey what's another quarter mill? By this stage, my collective debts exceeded the value of my assets by more than €16 million!

The worst thing about rapid success is just how painful and acute it all feels when things start to go in reverse. My head was full of regrets - all those decisions I took without a care in the world were coming back to haunt me.

But worse than all the financial headaches was the damage it did at home with the stress and strain taking its toll on our marriage. By 2011, we had separated and I was living alone in the Middle East franticly searching for investors who could turn things around.

During this period, I would spend weeks away from my children attempting to convince uninterested investors that my projects were unique and special when in reality the only things unique and special were the precious moments I was missing with my children. I started beating myself up for letting this happen and just when I thought things couldn't get any worse I received an email from my bank notifying me of their intention to implement what they called a *Full rental sweep.*

The implications of that email were felt immediately. Like flipping a switch, every penny of my income was now gone. In a few weeks' time I would not be able to afford my rent.

It's often only when you hit rock bottom that you begin to regain clarity and focus. I began to realise I had nowhere left to hide - the facade of success I had built myself had been stripped away. Reflecting on the journey, I realised I had been through the five stages of grief - from denial, to anger, to the what ifs of bargaining, to depression and finally to the point where I now found myself - acceptance.

I decided it was time to change the script.

Like flipping another switch, I decided I would take complete ownership for my failures. As much as I wanted to blame the big bad nasty world or the global financial crisis for my situation. It was not to blame: I was. I owned up to the fact I was the one who failed to keep my ego and emotions in check, nobody had forced me to borrow all that money and nobody had forced me to do all of those deals. It was at that moment that I regained control over my life.

Taking ownership for your situation is incredibly empowering. In that instant, I was transformed from being a victim with no control, to being back in the driver's seat. When you believe that life happens for you, not to you, good things start to happen. It's like an awakening, you realise that nobody is coming to rescue you and that the only person with the power to turn things around is you. In that moment any shame and regret I had about the past disappeared.

I felt excited by all the possibilities, like a movie script writer with a blank page in front of him, only this movie was my life and that blank page represents what I was going to do next. I took out my journal and started taking stock of the situation. I still had valuable assets that nobody could take away from me like my skills and my network, both critical to rebuilding a career. But what I also had was hard-earned experiences that gave me a unique insight into things all too often hidden from view.

More important still was the fact I had my health, both physical and mental - something I no longer took for granted having survived an unnatural level of stress and having witnessed up close, not once but twice, the awful impact of suicide by a family member and its aftermath on the loved ones left behind. Perhaps if I shared my insights I could help others avoid some of the mistakes and maybe even save lives. I found strength in giving my experience a meaning and purpose. Far from trying to conceal my failures I would embrace them and felt a sense of responsibility to share my story and its valuable lessons.

Remember, it's not your failures that define you, it's how you respond to failures that defines you as a person. It's how you get back up and how you choose to show up going forward. I have since recalibrated many of my goals in life. Whilst wealth and financial success are still a goal they are no longer the goal. I have made health a priority with the simple aim of being the fittest person I know and I set myself regular stretch goals and challenges accordingly.

Keen to challenge myself mentally too, I found that pushing myself out of my comfort zone opened new doors to opportunity. I joined Toastmasters with the aim of improving my public speaking and am today an international speaker, a skill I've developed to share my story with a larger audience, to that end, watch this space.

Today, some 12 years on, I view life as a tremendous adventure and a never-ending work in progress. I feel blessed to have the love and support of my wonderful fiancé Ilga and I could not be prouder of my three teenage daughters, Amber, Ashley and Alicia. I was also blessed with two more children, Erica and Dominic. I cherish the opportunity to watch them grow up with the love and guidance of their three older sisters.

They are my true legacy.

About Gavin J Gallagher

Gavin is an Irish property investor, entrepreneur and international speaker. A workplace expert with a degree in architecture, he designs and develops highly productive business environments. As Director of Earlsfort Group he runs East Point Business Park, an award 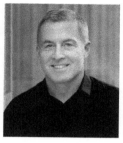 winning office campus that is home to more than 50 large multinational technology companies.

As host of podcast Behind The Facade, he explores the often overlooked but critically important mental and emotional game governing success in real estate. Reflecting on his career highs and lows, Gavin takes deep dives into the mindset, behaviours and the strategies essential to thrive in the property sector.

Building on the popularity of his podcast and in keeping with his mission to steer young investors away from the many of the pitfalls he encountered on his own journey, Gavin will publish his first book in 2021. For further details, see links below.

Contact Gavin J Gallagher

Website: https://gavinjgallagher.com/go

Podcast: https://anchor.fm/gavinjgallagher

Other Links: https://linktr.ee/gavinjgallagher

No One Thing

Speranza Holloway

Once upon a time I was a serial dieter. I spent 20 years of my life yo-yoing from one diet to the next as I believed being skinny was the missing thing I needed to feel complete. A new fad diet would come along and it would fire me up into a flurry of excitement, because each time I thought this diet would be the one to *make me skinny*. The obsessive dieting replaced the destructive and rebellious behaviour of my yout and marriage and two children had put the brakes on the crazy stuff!

Whichever way it manifested, the truth is, my chaotic behaviour was an attempt to fill the void caused by deep pain from a turbulent childhood. I had a husband who loves me, two amazing children, a lovely home, financial stability and lots of wonderful friends. But I felt unfulfilled without any understanding of why. I was unfit, overweight and constantly struggling with low self-esteem and I obsessed over finding the diet that would fix it. The obsessive cycle of dieting and failing left me exhausted, broken and filled with resentment. All my energy was channelled into licking my wounds. I focused on past traumas and let that narrative mould me.

Then things took a darker turn.

Over a two-year period my parents both became unwell, needed to move into a care home, became seriously ill, and died within six months of each other. I was suddenly and continuously immersed in my relationship with my parents, past and present, and I didn't have a single tool to cope emotionally. Engulfed by conflicting feelings of intense grief, despair and confusion, I was a complete mess.

Whilst packing up my family home and going through my parents' belongings, I pondered who they were and the impact of my upbringing on my current life, and I made the choice to be grateful for some parts and change others. I, my husband and my children deserved to have a well-rounded human being in their lives and I knew in my heart I wanted that too. I was grieving, but I did recognise it as the opportunity to make a clean break from the past and start afresh.

When I heard about a self-development networking group I decided to attend, despite being petrified. After attending that first meeting alone I was like a dog with a bone!!

I relentlessly returned to the group. Open-minded and curious, intently listening to the inspirational speakers and creaming off what I needed, I asked myself questions and absorbed the recommended resources too. Then the magic started to happen, and my life began to turn around! I began to feel empowered, positive and optimistic. With my new-found confidence I ran... 5k... 10k... a half marathon then the unimaginable: a MARATHON!!

With every new step I was scared and filled with self-doubt; running, open water swimming, fire walking, events and courses, but I recognised that the nerves would push me out of my comfort zone and fuel the change. I achieved my slim badge, gained good health, fitness and a sense of mental wellness. My most significant source of joy now comes from the ability to stride through life with my head held high because every push to a new achievement gave my confidence a massive boost.

The life-changing lesson I have learned on my mind-body transformation is the realisation that NO ONE THING was going to fix me. NO ONE THING you apply, buy or buy into is the answer to your problem, whatever the problem. Once you drop the ingrained belief in the one fix cure, you'll be free to get to work and power through the steps it takes to feel and look incredible.

I know you know, because you're not daft, that a balanced diet and regular exercise are essential to healthy living.

So, why is it that many of us fail to be consistent and get results?

In the past, I would agree every time someone would say *It's not rocket science, just eat less and exercise more,* but I never understood what was stopping me putting this principle into practice. To achieve your goal of looking incredible and feeling on top of the world (you'd like that right?), it's essential to conquer that crazy bonkers mind of yours.

Looking after your well-being and mental health is an integral part of that transition. But where to start?

I've discovered that to get the ball rolling we need to focus on changing our perception; a little re-education; and developing a handful of new habits or rituals. Then the non-negotiable exercise and nutritious eating will slip in seamlessly. I'm not unique. I don't have more will power than you. I've just taught myself a new approach.

Here's the thing - it's not your fault if you've never gained your tip-top health badge. It's incredibly challenging to look outside of the box when your perceived solutions are so profoundly embedded and based on a lifetime of the hard sell (holding back on a rant here).

So, what do I mean by changing your perception?

It's taking one perceived way of thinking and injecting an alternative one to take its place. One step at a time, one belief at a time, until we have a shiny new approach. I've been working on the *Project Me* for a handful of years now and have devised a process filled with fresh new ideas.

Here is one of the examples to get you started and give you a taste of what I mean. Before you throw this one out of the park, remember the open-minded approach I took when I was looking for answers and how it benefited me.

Step one, cease blaming others. Blaming others holds you back in the past. When you live in the past, it is incredibly difficult to progress because it consumes all your thoughts. Positive action cannot take place if your thoughts aren't clear. If the water is muddy it's harder to dive in. I understand that painful experiences happen every day and you cannot control whether or not others behave in a hurtful way.

You may even be unaware that you are playing the blame game but I'd like you to consider adopting this approach: STOP focusing on the actions of others and instead, focus on what action you can take (whether it's your wicked step mum or the chap that cut you up on the round-about).

It's not your fault, but it is your responsibility. Taking responsibility makes it easier to take action, which is an essential part of making a positive change.

Basic healthy eating is at the heart of obtaining and maintaining a beautiful, strong, lean, fit mind and body.

Here is a practical habit that you can put in place to get you started and keep you on track. Daily food prepping is one simple, practical action you can take that will have a massive impact on what you consume in the day. The purpose is to grow a strong, healthy eating bias by conditioning a ritual through repetition. There is no taking away, just adding, as depriving yourself is a one-way ticket to failure.

Start by writing two lists, one of the fruit you like, one of the vegetables you like. This process clarifies and acts as a reminder that there are healthy foods you are willing to eat and bins any negativity you may have around this food group.

Then, every morning prep your food for the busiest part of the day, including grab-and-go snacks and a salad lunch made up from the list. Ensure your salad is tasty by adding, for example, extra virgin olive oil, sea salt, or any item that has no more than four ingredients, clean and additive free. Do this every day to condition yourself to the simple flavours until you can't live without them and you've brainwashed yourself to improve your diet! I know this is possible because I've cracked it. I'm a former Cookie Monster who now eats clean the majority of the time.

Finally, a warning about whinging when you are eating: I'm expecting you to create happy, upbeat energy when the healthy food is entering your mouth. Even if you are telling yourself a white lie, repeat it until you form a positivity habit.

I love the metaphor of a jigsaw puzzle for living your best life. You lay down one piece, one action, ONE THING at a time. Each individual piece comes together to build a whole picture. You never rush it. You ponder and quiz every single piece to place it correctly and it's thrilling when you get it right. Occasionally you mess up, and it takes some wiggling and manoeuvring to set the piece free. You start again, but you never give up; because your eye is on the whole picture, your best life.

Live your best life now, because when that puzzle is complete you can work on another, one piece at a time.

About Speranza Holloway

Speranza, is a mind fitness coach, the founder of *Mind Body Slim* and the author/creator of *No One Thing*.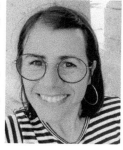

She started her mind-body transformation journey back in 2017, although from a young age, has had an inkling that life had so much more to offer Before the journey was started she struggled to walk up the stairs and now can't imagine a life without marathon running.

Speranza feels so passionate about getting people moving that she set up the running group *Check me in, Check me out Run Club* and is thrilled to witness the participants joy from their achievements.

Previously on anti-depressants, she adopted a fix herself approach to health and wellness and has exceeded what she set out to achieve.

Her do something for humanity mission has led to a new career path, helping others through emotional awareness and implementing change one small step at a time.

Contact Speranza Holloway

https://linktr.ee/Speranzaholloway

speranzamindfitnesscoach@outlook.com

I Can See Clearly Now!

R. G. Wysocki

Welcome to my story, a story of someone who seemed doomed to fail in life but discovered later his real purpose to live in abundance and happiness. My hope is that this story will uplift you, especially in these phenomenally uncertain times. Most of you will have limiting beliefs but you also have exceptional abilities, something to share, to contribute through living inside out from our heart.

I grew up as an only child from a remarried couple. Both parents were employed, busy and working and their earnings were comfortable, although they didn't own anything as I learned later as an adult. They spent excessively going out and visiting places around the world.

I guess we were considered middle class. I was a dreamer, naive, spoiled, lacking success in school to the disdain of my parents. I believed that it was not my fault but rather due to the fact that my parents travelled and changed country every 3-4 years. Somehow it generated a doubt in me. Without any roots, I was considered a foreigner everywhere we moved to with difficulties integrating. What I missed most were lasting friendships. I didn't have any. This had a strong effect on my future development.

In my last teenage year about to graduate from High School I lost my mother to cancer. It was so sudden that I didn't even realize it. I was desperate, almost suicidal, judged by the way I was driving to the hospital to see her one last time. At that point she was the only love in my life and I blamed myself for many years about not showing up, sharing my love, saying simple words, reflecting my feelings and expressing my gratitude.

"Between what is said and not meant, and what is meant and not said, most of love is gone."
Kahlil Gibran

After graduation - which I had to sit and pass alone as the death of my mother delayed the normal exams schedule for me - came a time of unconscious wandering through life. I was 19 with no idea or vision what to do with my life. I was depressed, doubting and blaming myself for not being enough.

That summer I enrolled into a student trip through Scandinavia. Driving through the Fjords with their deep, dark blue waters was a beauty of nature that I couldn't even perceive. On this trip I discovered a beautiful song from Johnny Nash, *I Can See Clearly Now* which clearly was the exact opposite of my being and made me even more depressed. That trip in no way uplifted me and when I came back I started reading Nietzsche and Dostoevsky who came perfectly in time driving my self-love and acceptance further down when starting my Philosophy studies.

It didn't last long.

I quit Philosophy because I felt more miserable than ever,

always blaming myself and convinced that I was a loser who couldn't achieve anything.

"Our life is what our thoughts make it."
Marcus Aurelius, Roman Emperor

I was living on a subsidy granted by the international organization that my mother worked for and which would continue if I pursued my studies. Being conditioned through my parents lavish lifestyle, I bought myself a big car and suddenly I had many friends. It was financially difficult at times because I was overspending due to the lack of financial education and so I took on some side jobs. Came a day, after failing in Philosophy, for which I don't exactly remember the circumstances, some friends dragged me into studies of Economics to take responsibility and allow myself a decent future. During these studies was a sudden click in my mind. I realized I was really on my own, nobody to save me, and if I wanted to live a worry-free life I needed to make money. This became my purpose. I started to invest in the stock market, buying stocks in companies as advised by my bank.

Back in the early 1980s was the worst time to get into stocks back when fixed income products would have made a greater return. I learnt my lesson and decided never to listen to a banker again as they know nothing - at least apparently not more than me. I then picked up specialized magazines in technical and fundamental analysis, all of the research and orders were paper-based back then. Compared to nowadays, it wasn't easy as you had to walk to your bank or call them to place an order and wait until the next day for the outcome.

Today it is so easy, all orders and transactions are online

commission-free or only marginal. With some research, reading and basic principles implemented, there are no excuses today to not be successful.

"Take the first step in faith. You don't have to see the whole staircase, just take the first step."
Martin Luther King Jr.

After graduating, I was barely financially self-sufficient so I wanted to join the banking sector to learn how to reach my purpose, to become wealthy and to gain social recognition.

A first unsuccessful job ensued then I got lucky being hired by the Belgian subsidy of an American Investment Bank, JP Morgan. I landed the job not so much because of my not really brilliant studies but more due to my language skills, acquired through all our moves. Following a few years of learning how the bank operated, working mostly with American Institutional Investors, I was offered the opportunity to move to New York in 1990, hence being closer to them and avoiding time zone differences.

"Focus on where you want to be and not where you were, or where you are."
Anthony Robbins

For me, the 1990s were the golden years - meeting celebrities, flying Concorde, having my apartment in New York, a lavish lifestyle, all I desired when I was younger, right? But ...

Somehow, I was missing something, but what?

The results were there, undeniable, the Dow Jones[1] climbed 370% in the decade from October 1990 to December 1999 while my clients performed over three times better. So what was wrong? Shouldn't I be happy? I had what I desired so much when younger, what was missing?

I need to mention that while working hard and earning well I got married which didn't last long due to my incapacity to truly love and cherish that relationship. Yet another failure.

It became obvious to me that I wasn't fulfilled despite my professional success. I realized that my life was empty, everything I touched felt superficial, unnecessary, excessive and depressing.

> *"Success is not the key to happiness,*
> *happiness is the key to success."*
> Albert Schweitzer

I finally realized that I was living outside in, wearing a mask, emulating someone I was not, all of this to get social acceptance and recognition. I created over time what Carl G. Jung names a *Persona*[2], showing a person I am not, but which myself and others think I am.

I needed to dig deeper.

At that stage I decided to go back to my roots. I quit the bank and moved back to Belgium where I had the most lasting memories by far, good and bad. I didn't take up another job immediately. I had this urgent need to understand where my suffering came from, so I started consulting a psychologist. We went deeper together, we went through what Anthony Robbins calls the Dickens Process, uncovering your limiting beliefs and how they will further dictate your future if you don't change them. I discovered that I had a dark side, the part I was suppressing in me, my unconscious belief that I cannot experience true love. It became clear to me that it all goes back to my relationship with my mother and her sudden death and all the unspoken and undone that I blamed myself for. What a discovery some 20 years later! The therapy helped me immensely, gradually putting an end to my suffering, and so I began a new life with a different mindset, freeing me slowly from my limiting beliefs and guiding me towards love and appreciation.

"Every problem is a gift; without problems we would not grow."
Anthony Robbins

Since then I met my wife and we've been together now for 23 years, raised two children and live a life of abundance.

It hasn't always been easy, there were ups and downs. In the summer of 2008, we left Jamaica after living there for five years, our move to Italy occurred in the middle of the 2008 Financial crisis culminating into the bankruptcy of Lehman Brothers. I had no online access to hedge my investments, I almost lost everything. It was a painful moment but also I knew that this will not last and create a new opportunity to bounce back. I basically got greedy and now it was pay-time, I took the lesson and what really saved me was the love we shared as a family.

We learned to nurture our relationship even more from the many Anthony Robbins events that we attended. We learned so much about ourselves and our relationship through questioning openly our thoughts, words and actions.

Life is a gift as Anthony Robbins always says, a new day is a gift. So many people are denied the chance to make a difference with another day. Imagine today is your last day. Would you continue doing what you always did or would this thought help you to take a new, more fulfilling path?

My main mantra today is to appreciate more and expect less, even in adverse situations. We all are students of life and our willingness to learn on our way undoubtedly will make a difference in us and the world we live in.

And today, I love to listen to the song from Johnny Nash that in the past inflicted me so much suffering. Today, I am on my way and there are no obstacles on the way to my best life.

"Success is doing what you want to do, when you want, where you want, with whom you want, as much as you want."
Anthony Robbins

References

1. The Dow Jones is a US stock market index that measures the stock performance of 30 large companies listed on US stock exchanges, Source: macrotrends.net, Dow Jones from October 1990 to December 1999

2. Carl G. Jung, The Archetypes and the Collective Unconscious, Volume 9, part I of The Collected Works, Princetown University Press, 1990, p. 123.

About R.G. Wysocki

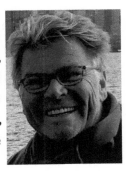

Rainer G. Wysocki is an investor and philanthropist who has worked with JP Morgan in Brussels and New York, managing multimillion dollar institutional accounts. Throughout his career he always focused on his clients' best interests, achieved superior results and hence entertained a faithful customer base.

After his banking career he decided to join the Financial Software sector where he took on different roles to expand their businesses, he ended his career at Hyperion Solutions as Director for Belgium and Luxembourg before retiring early in 2003.

Since then he focuses mainly on his family, his wife, their two kids and the many dogs and wherever he lives he always tries to help the less fortunate. His and his wife's latest project at heart is the creation of an orphan foundation.

As he says himself: "Comes a time in your life, a time to give back."

Superpower Confidence

Steph Robin

"Confidence is a preference."
Damon Albarn, Blur

Confidence is the magic ingredient that supercharges your mindset and actions, rocketing you towards your fully lived life. If you are in a confident state you dream bigger, think bigger, commit bigger, act bigger, love bigger… for you, your family plus your organisation and teams. Confidence is a muscle. We all have it, but for some it can be ignored and neglected. In the same way that we can strengthen the muscles in our body by working out and stretching, we can also improve our confidence by taking the same approach of consistency and focus.

Confidence allows you to look at yourself, others and your environment with positivity and optimism. That things have been good, opportunities have been seized, growth has been achieved. Confidence also enables you to be comfortable with your failures with the knowledge that learning comes from any attempt to move forward and grow, regardless of the end result. Confidence is your superpower, like a powerful autopilot, constantly and subtly guiding you to make and execute the right choices.

Confidence is not arrogance. It's strength under-pinned by both certainty and humility. It is swelled by evidence of success and progression, no-matter how inelegant. A confident mindset enables you to see the value you bring to yourself and others but is grounded by the knowledge that your practice is always evolving and you have much to learn as well as to share.

Why bother? Let's pause all this positive talk for a minute and consider what life is like when your confidence has been dented. The superpower weakens, doubt creeps in, options narrow. Too many dings left unchecked can result in crisis of confidence. From this place, the world seems smaller; doors close, allies disappear, ideas dry up and hope seems lost.

How do I know? I've been there.

In the middle of a high-flying career that had taken me all over the world starting businesses, I found myself suddenly on a different trajectory. I'd exited a job that hadn't gone well and found myself completely lost trying to find my way back into employment. I'd lost faith in not only my ability to be effective but also that I even knew what it was that I was good at in the first place. Recruitment consultants didn't know how to place me, applications went unanswered and when I did get an interview it seemed quickly that I was applying for the wrong role. I remember clearly, painfully getting a rejection from a phone interview mere minutes after I hung up. That really stung. It was brutal. Rejection hurts. My world of work was getting smaller.

Funny thing is, at the same time I was getting physically bigger. I'd lost my sense of direction, I had nothing clear to aim for, I had no reason to be in shape. I just wanted comfort and to remain still as anything else was just too difficult and whatever I tried wasn't resulting in success. This turn of events dismantled my confidence.

I had enough fight left in me to know I needed help and sought the advice of incredible coaches and mentors. Leveraging powerful personal insights, direction and focus I was able to not only recharge my confidence superpower but use it to change my career, reclaim my health and start my own business. From a more confident position I was bold enough to realise that I was wasting my time applying for jobs with a CV and I needed to carve out my own speciality and serve that fully as opposed to trying to fit into somebody else's mould.

Take it from me, losing confidence can be like death from a thousand cuts. You don't feel the first few, but if you don't stem the bleeding you can be in deep trouble before you really know it.

Want the good news? You and you alone are in charge of your confidence and you can absolutely build it back up to full superpower. You can learn to protect and grow it. The wonderful thing is that this journey back up from the depths swells your confidence even more. It presents evidence that you are strong, that you are capable of winning, of over-coming the odds, of being able to navigate difficult times.

So, how do we curate this precious confidence?

There are three areas of focus:

1. Program your superpower. Think of it like an autopilot that makes your decisions based on data not emotions. Log the data that demonstrates unarguably that you are good and have done good things.

2. Develop a rigorous data-driven defence that deflects sabotage attempts from you and others.

3. Introduce and maintain nourishing habits that fuel and sustain your confidence and present more data to show you are a winner.

Let's start with programming your *superpower*.

Find a quiet moment and a quiet place to reflect. Collect the events and results that demonstrate your effectiveness across the full range of your life. In work, in relationships, in your financial health and your physical health. What are the data points that show you matter? You will find the list is longer than you expected and when you really get into flow you will find it hard to stop. If you're struggling to get started ask family, friends and colleagues to share what you are good at, what your finest moments have been. As a minimum you must fill a full page of A4. If you don't do this, you are underpowering your superpower.

Take a moment to check in how you feel after doing this exercise. What's your inner voice saying? Are you standing a little taller? Is there a smile curling on your lips? It's OK to whisper secretly to yourself that you are actually a badass, a humble badass of course! What we've done here is to program our superpower with facts. Presented with the true story, our minds can begin to see us as capable and deserving.

Let's get ugly.

We will now focus on developing a rigorous *data-driven defence* of our confidence. This confidence muscle can be strained or torn by the actions of others. It's important to know when your confidence has been impacted so that then you can take action to pump it up again. What are the things that can chip away at your confidence? Not to be dramatic, but threats can come from many angles. Toxic personal relationships, challenging situations in the workplace, a few days or weeks of not making progress ... belief dips and confidence is eroded. Want the good news? This is entirely normal and experienced by even the most successful performers. Think of sportspeople with a loss of form, CEOs that bring out a product that misfires, musicians with a flop album. It's not about never dipping - it's about knowing what to do to get back on track.

This is where your superpower protects you. In the face of unkind words or awkward fails, the data in your superpower presents the truth and can be used to debunk any fake news. True confident strength comes not from running away from your critics or problems, but from meeting them head on and having a grown-up debate that presents your case for the defence. Yes, you might have made a whopper of a mistake, but does that erase years of success and right choices? What would you say?

Make friends with your cringe and see it as a learning asset. As a young manager, I got disastrous feedback from a manager during an appraisal. A comment stating I was unconfident in front of people wasn't said in the face to face meeting but snuck in on the official form that was shared across the management team. I was crushed and utterly embarrassed.

Shame kills confidence. I allowed it to become a self-limiting belief and allowed it to remain so for years, holding me back from applying for jobs and approaching people. It only evaporated it with the aid of a more supportive manager who helped me present the true data. Kindly interrogate information in order to process it with perspective and categorise it correctly.

This debate takes courage and courage takes strength, so to be in the best shape to grow and defend your confidence you have to look after yourself.

Develop habits that show you matter. These habits give you the best chance of sustaining your physical and mental health. These conditions are uniquely personal so once again find space and time to identify the habits that unlock your success. Go back to a time when you were really flying, feeling good, delivering brilliantly. What was in your life? How did you get energy? Who was with you? What are the environmental and habitual clues to your success? Know what they are and then commit to making them part of your life again. I will share some of mine and it's a simple mix of gratitude journaling, creating headspace and getting daily movement. If you are ever feeling off for more than a couple of days in a row, check in to see if you are still practicing your nourishing habits.

As a special bonus I'm going to add a fourth secret ingredient to super-charge confidence.

Set yourself *outrageous goals*. Ones that you immediately regret making but a target that requires you to change your mindset and habits in order to achieve it.

For me that was a triathlon.

As an overweight and over-40 something I had no right to be signing up for an activity that requires squeezing into a wetsuit. Especially as that was only one part of a trio of physical discomforts. I didn't prepare as much as a I should have for the water and was extremely close to a panic attack as I got the furthest away from shore. However, my superpower kicked in, reminded my panic that I was physically fit and stubbornly determined and that was all the evidence I needed to calm down and swim on. My intense relief saw me flee out of the water and crush the bike and run and now I have another data point powering up my confidence superpower.

You now know the importance of strengthening and protecting your confidence superpower.

The ultimate demonstration of your certainty is to use your strength to help others. Take a moment each day to reach out to someone and boost their confidence. Give them a gift to load into their superpower and help them realise the life they dare to dream of, unlocked by confidence.

About Steph Robin

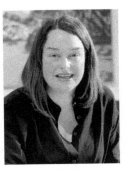

Coaching with Steph focuses on super-charging confidence by developing positive mindset and behaviours. Working with both individuals and teams, Steph's coaching style is relentlessly energetic, practical and obsessed with progress. Her down to earth approach leverages her 20-year career in Big Data and Digital launching and growing businesses and teams around the world. She's also living proof that you can change your life, turning around a dangerously unhealthy lifestyle and overcoming redundancy.

Steph has led global operations for data science consultancies working across retail, consumer goods, entertainment and digital media and for clients including Tesco, Mars, Macy's and Sky. Her work has taken her all over the world from the UK to the USA and India.

In addition to Executive Coaching, Steph provides consulting services to large organisations seeking to futureproof leadership behaviours, mindsets and workspaces to deliver a world class employee experience.

Contact Steph Robin

hello@stephrobin.com

www.stephrobin.com

The Story Of Here And There

Sumaya Alshamsi

I remember when I was a kid watching an episode of *Sesame Street*. In that episode, two big monsters were trying to teach the little monster the words: *here* and *there*.

The first big monster points at the spot where he was standing with the little monster and told him, *That's here*; and then points at another spot where the other big monster stands and said, *That's there*.

The little monster squealed, *I want to be there* and ran as fast as he could and when he reached the other spot, he asked enthusiastically, *Am I there now?*

The second big monster said, *No, now you are here*.

The little monster was confused and asked, *Where is there? I want to be there*.

The second adult monster pointed to where the first adult monster was standing and said, *There!*

So, the little monster ran back to the first spot, again.

You can guess that the little monster ran back and forth between the two spots.

Of course, he will never reach *there*, because each *there* he reaches will turn into *here*.

And this can be true for a lot of people who are searching desperately for happiness, frantically running everywhere and clearly looking in all the wrong places.

It's just like a mirage in the desert. It looks like water but the more you chase it, the further away it seems, and the thirstier you become. And the tragedy is you will never find it because ultimately it's an illusion.

It's like the world around us.

Our reality is a reflection of who we are. Each person's values, beliefs, decisions and memories form a glass that we see the world through. It is so much like a Snapchat filter that can turn any face into an angel, clown or a dog!

Changing your reality and the world around you requires a simple and brave decision but it requires you to begin by looking inside yourself to find your truth.

Gandhi summed it up perfectly by saying, *Be the change you want to see in the world.*

Einstein explained it by saying, *The most important decision we make is whether we believe we live in a friendly or hostile universe.*

One of the most powerful tools is to write a *gratitude list,* every day. Things you are grateful for. Writing a gratitude list will train your mind to focus on things that make you happy.

You might be grateful for the obvious benefits in your life.

Or you might be just as grateful for the small, benign, everyday things that sustain, fulfil and delight that can easily get overlooked. Simple things that you take for granted.

Koreans call it *sohwakhaeng* - a simple but certain happiness. Essentially, it is finding a certain happiness in small things. Appreciating the magical moments in ordinary daily life such as the warmth of sun light on your skin, or the aroma of freshly ground coffee. Finding these simple moments of happiness add up to making a beautiful and more fulfilling life.

Ichi-go ichi-e is a Japanese phrase I learnt last year. It means one time, one meeting and is a cultural concept of valuing and treasuring every moment. Each moment is a once in a lifetime experience. Every second of your life that passes will never come back.

The questions I ask myself every day are:

- What if today was the last day of my life?
- What if I never have this experience again?
- Or meet this person again?

Another cultural concept in Japan is *kaizan* which means *change for the better*. It is about constant improvement or always challenging yourself.

Simply, no one knows what you are able to do, except you. No one knows what your soul truly desires and what makes your heart sing, except you.

If you do something you know that is not aligned with your values - no matter how many compliments you get from everyone - you will never feel or be fulfilled.

Trying to meet the expectations of others or being driven by the need for approval will only leave your soul starving. No matter how hard you try to fit in - just like the wrong piece of a puzzle - you never will.

It is better to live an imperfect life as your true identity than to try to live a fake perfect life where you tick all the boxes for the sake of ticking boxes. Or to please others in a way that you recognise as neither healthy nor positive.

As the Dr Seuss quote says, *Why fit in when you were born to stand out?*

So, let go of all the false identities and the labels you have collected in your life. Face your past. It's not supposed to haunt you or shame you. All the mistakes you have made are supposed to be learning experiences. Failure is normal. You're supposed to fail... to win. Use your past to fuel your passion and push you forward to live your best life.

In the game of life, it's not how you start, it's how you finish the game that matters.

Maybe you can even make your own rules to win your own game of life. Or to simply do your best.

As Mark Twain said, *The two most important days in your life are the day you are born ... and the day you find out why.*

About Sumaya Alshamsi

Sumaya Alshamsi is a dreamer, certified life coach and a motivational speaker.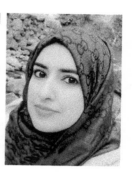

She is on a mission to help women find their voices and speak their truth.

Her dream is to leave a sparkle of joy everywhere she goes and to make the world a happier place

Contact Sumaya Alshamsi

sralshamsi106@gmail.com

Instagram: dance_with_life2020

The Pursuit Of Confidence

Clare Honeyfield

The most common thing other women say to me is, "Wow, I don't know how you do that! You must be so confident!"

Well, let me tell you, it has not always been so.

Building my confidence has been a slow and steady practice and I occasionally fall off the confidence wagon and feel *not good enough*. But you know what? I always get back on and carry on, regardless. If there is one thing I have learned in life, it is not to listen to my own self doubt.

As a mum of four, I only started exercising formally when my youngest was a teenager. Somehow, in between businesses, a home and the mum taxi I just never found time.

I bought a book, something about running a 10k in six months. Then came my first half marathon (I'd run ultra marathons as a teenager but hadn't run for decades – I could hardly run for the bus!)

With the running, came a new confidence and a new body of course. And with the new body (which I must say is ever changing in all directions) came a new found love of dressing up, having fun, dancing and getting into performance arts. I then began what I would describe as an all-out journey to myself. Often, actually travelling further away from myself rather than closer to myself, oddly.

I got back into going to music festivals, finding every crew job possible at Glastonbury, trained in pole dancing, became a cancan dancer for a few summers, started learning trapeze, silks, rope and hoop, and ultimately, trained as a yoga teacher.

There was never a *plan* as such, I just really threw myself into the pursuit of me. I think having had so many years of being focussed on others made me kind of self obsessed, but not necessarily in a bad way.

When I first started Stroud farmers' market, at the age of 36, I was so shy that I didn't want to be in the photograph of the official opening with Jasper Conran and Isabella Blow. Luckily, the photographer from the local paper insisted. I had no idea how to pose for a photo and felt awkward and ugly. I don't feel proud to say that, but I felt unattractive for many years. I just really didn't know what to do with myself. Literally.

I've had to overcome feelings of being a fraud, chronic imposter syndrome, whilst stood on the stage of the annual farmers' market conference talking about marketing, whilst picking up business awards over decades, and sometimes when getting out of bed in the morning.

The one thing I learned over this time is just to keep showing up, keeping doing the next right thing, to follow my passions and not to listen to my inner dialogue, which is mostly the irrelevant wittering on of societal norms I had picked up along the way.

I have had to have a good long hard look at myself, and then I've had to create some new neural pathways, super charge my cells with water and improved nutrition, push myself to do things I don't feel confident doing, but love and want to do. Isn't that a curious thing?

For the first two years of training aerial, I was constantly putting myself down in my mind. Then one day, I just told the rest of the class that I tell myself *I'm no good, too old, will never be a strong as everyone else,* and it's like a bit of alchemy happened in that moment, because from that time onwards, I have experienced nothing but joy and connection in that class.

I guess sometimes we just have to grass ourselves up to our peers. Saying something out loud is so powerful and somehow dissipates the energy of a deeply held limiting belief.

As well as getting fitter and stronger, through various means from hiring a personal trainer to attending outdoor boot camp classes, I have attended trainings, listened to audio books, devoured podcasts and surrounded myself with people I aspire to be like - people who contribute, serve, better themselves and get in touch with their inner super hero.

I've learned that life is a series of decisions, of choices and of possibilities. There have been times when I've felt discouraged, overwhelmed and lost, but I look back at these times as periods of great growth. I have learned not to be discouraged. Life owes us nothing, there are no guarantees. We are here for a moment and then we are just a memory. It's not about becoming someone great, it's about experiencing the greatness within ourselves. It's about feeling good about stuff we've done, it's about contributing and getting out of our own way.

I treat myself as a welcome guest in my own home. Feed myself plenty of fresh, organic high vibrational plant based foods. Drink plenty of clean water.

My home is a sanctuary of peace and tranquility. I surround myself with beauty, clean often and let go of clutter I don't need. My home is a place I love to return to, a place of peace and of safety in a crazy noisy world.

I have learned to run myself lovely bubble baths, listen to my favourite music, listen to new music, light candles and have lovely smells to make me feel good. I like to keep a collection of essential oils in the bathroom.

I start each day with peace and gratitude, give myself some space, enjoy my shower, and aim to be in the moment. I wear clothes which make me feel good. Replace my socks and underwear when they wear old, treat myself to nice things, well made things, things made by people who get a good deal.

I've learned that the world can be a loud and sometimes vexatious place. Everyone has something to say. Everyone has an opinion, everyone likes to give advice. I have learned to listen to my own inner voice, my inner guru, my higher self, the universe flowing through me. This is probably the most valuable skill I can hone in my life, I think.

If I had to give myself advice, this would be it:

Always push yourself to be a better person, to add more value, to give more, to think outside of society's rather limiting boxes, and to finish what you have started. Keep showing up, never give up, believe in yourself and know that those who are successful in life are those who are consistently brave with their actions.

Make your bed in the morning. That way you start each day having achieved something already.

Always be courageous with your decisions, but surround yourself with people who have your back, so that when things don't work out, they are there to carry you. And be that person who other people can rely on too.

Learn to meditate, learn to be with yourself, and learn the value of stillness. Then you have the resources to bring that calm into any situation you find yourself in.

Don't beat yourself up when you do something that disappoints you. You are not perfect and there is no such thing as perfection in life.

Never underestimate the value of chilled filtered water, morning coffee, a wild swim with friends, picnics, firelight and laughter for a happy life.

When you look in the mirror, say kind things to yourself. Look into your eyes and see the beauty which resides in your soul. If you could see yourself as others see you, you would see your perfection, your utter lovability and your great potential.

Only hang out with people who are a tonic for your soul, who light you up, make you feel warm inside and with whom you feel connection and importantly, safety.

And laugh often.

Always try to be kind and generous, even though it is not fashionable, because it will make you feel better about yourself. Give what you can afford to give but don't tolerate takers in your inner circle.

Find yourself a practice, so that when you are tempted to seek out darkness, you can return to a place of balance within yourself and you can avoid harming yourself or others along the way. It doesn't matter what the practice is, but keep seeking until you find it. And then make it part of you.

Try not to judge too much or when you do judge, wear your judgment like a light cloak you can discard at any time.

Most of all, try to leave the world a better place, give more than you have received, and be the person you would have liked in your life. Because then you have everything you need to live your best life.

About Clare Honeyfield

Clare Honeyfield was a founding director of the National Association of Farmers' Markets and founder of Stroud farmers' market which was launched by Isabella Blow and Jasper Conran in 1999. Going on to set up the first private farmers' market operating company outside London, her flagship event in 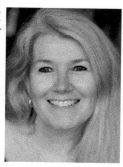 Stroud was the first weekly farmers' market outside the capital and remains the most awarded farmers' market in the UK. Clare was a cofounder of Gloucestershire Food Links and The Gloucestershire Association of Farmers' Markets.

Since 2012, Clare has been sole director of *The Made in Stroud Shop*, which she helped to set up as a makers cooperative with 25 members in December 2000. Now working with 160 makers, the shop runs as a successful multi award winning social enterprise and is a Plastic Free Champion.

Clare is a coach working with entrepreneurs and creatives, speaker, and writer.

Clare works as a consultant in ethical community retail.

Contact Clare Honeyfield

Clare Honeyfield Coach is on Instagram and Facebook

www.madeinstroud.co.uk

clare@madeinstroud.co.uk

Healing The Energies Within A Business

Yvette K. Smith

Quite a few years ago, I reached a crossroad in my life. My husband had recently gone through a tumultuous period in his business owing to the actions of his unscrupulous business partner and the partnership broke up. This obviously had a very devastating effect on us, on both a financial and emotional level. After the initial shock, catching our breath and taking a reality check, we took stock of our situation and decided that we needed a complete change of scenery to move forward, so we sold our house and moved back to the part of the country that we had grown up in. This had the added bonus of living close to my family once more and our children could grow up with their cousins.

Relocating to a completely different part of the country can be a difficult venture, both for parents and for children. The children have to get used to a whole new world without their familiar routines, make new friends and cope with being the outsiders for a while until they once again become firmly entrenched in their social life. As parents, our challenges were the same in part and different in others. The pressure was on to find decent schools, a new home which was pet-friendly as we had numerous dogs, to make new friends (as we enjoy having a healthy social life) and most importantly for my husband, to break new ground by connecting with strangers and making a completely new network of contacts in the business world so that he could once again start earning an income. It was tough going, but we tightened our belts, spent money only on essentials and he persevered until he began making inroads and work began to slowly flow in. Although we had family close by, it was still quite a lonely existence at the time but we managed to keep our spirits up and kept moving forward, one step at a time.

I come from a family of entrepreneurs and I'm very happy to say that my husband (who came from a family of hard working, but extremely risk averse parents) was ambitious enough to embrace the concept of entrepreneurship from very early on in our marriage. Consequently, he has always supported me by encouraging me to work for myself and so I have managed to do that for quite a large part of my working life.

One day, an opportunity crossed my path.

Initially, I was a tad reluctant to take it on board as it was a completely new industry for me and I was filled with some trepidation, but I eventually decided to take the bull by the horns and take over this small business and see where it would lead me. I still made a massive effort to be there for my children as much as possible and see to their needs as they were used to me working from home and therefore always being around, but it often meant that I worked late into the night until the wee small hours, trying to perfect systems and working on formulas on Excel spreadsheets, determined to make them all work before going to bed. If truth be told, I actually found it exciting and enjoyed it.

I grew my little business until I had a few smallish clients and one very large, lucrative client, many employees and a significant financial turnover. My business was running smoothly and I could now take a large amount of time off to spend with my family, apart from a few non-negotiable hours every week. Things were good until one day it became obvious that my large client was beginning to struggle to keep his business afloat. The economy was not great and there were many political agendas at play, that were beginning to have devastating effects on some of the larger companies as they struggled to keep their heads above water. The signs were all there. My client tried to keep afloat for as long as possible, but eventually he called a meeting with me. It seemed that he was so desperate that he was willing to renege on one of his financial agreements with me.

I had my ear to the ground and was aware of his intention.

Let me just say that he was a decent person but because he was so desperate to save as much of his company as possible and come out as financially strong as he could, he was grasping at straws and trying to claw back as much money as he could. So, long story short, I was faced with a similar scenario as someone who pays household insurance to a company for a year, but at the end of the year they have had no break-ins and therefore have not had to make any claims, so they then demand all their previous insurance payments be refunded to them. Fortunately, I had some leverage as I had only charged him half of my normal fees for the entire contract.

As it was, I had recently been introduced to energy medicine. I had been very stressed about the imminent loss of my biggest paying client and two different friends had recommended that I make an appointment with an energy healer that they were both seeing. After an initial appointment, with a couple of follow up appointments, I became so fascinated by the concept of using energy medicine to heal my mind and body that I began learning all about it.

I had only recently learnt the very basics of energy medicine when my business meeting was scheduled and had also come across the term, *Conflict Resolution*. This somehow seemed a fitting time to use my newly acquired skills to resolve this conflict in my business life.

I used a mind tool named MindScape to visualise a meeting between us, playing out the entire meeting and what questions either of us would ask as well as the answers that would result in an outcome that we could both agree upon and be happy with. I held this visual meeting twice before I attended the real-life meeting.

Twice, the client rescheduled the meeting but because I was using my mind tool, I was quite calm about it and on the day of the actual meeting, I implemented another method of energy medicine as I was driving to the meeting. I used a technique named *Tapping the Cortices*. This technique means (amongst other actions), tapping over the right and left brain at the same time to restore communication between both halves of the brain - the logical left brain and the creative right brain. I visualised myself tapping out the client's cortices, over and over and over again, during the entire 20-minute journey. My client, however, was running late and the ladies in the office looked at me with sympathy as they said that he was in such a foul mood that day, that they hoped that he wouldn't be too harsh with me.

So I sat there tapping away.

When he arrived, I was most surprised that his mood seemed quite mild and we proceeded to his office for a meeting that lasted only about 5-10 minutes in which he asked if he could talk first and I could ask questions after. I obviously agreed and he then proceeded to state almost exactly what I had anticipated in my visual meetings with him. I agreed to give him a refund of all monies that had not been used for the previous year, if he paid me three quarters of my normal fees, instead of the half that we had negotiated at the commencement of the contract. This meant that instead of insisting on my full fees, I still was giving him a quarter off, which he was appreciative of. In essence, it was mostly a restructuring of the monies and resulted in an acceptable outcome as we both gained some and lost some. It had been a good meeting and we parted with no animosity.

It was at this stage that I realised that energy medicine could most definitely help to heal not only our physical bodies, but our businesses as well. With the help of energy medicine, my business had come through relatively unscathed from a potentially cataclysmic scenario. From that point on, I concentrated more on my studies and qualified as a BodyTalk Practitioner, deciding that I would like to focus on helping businesses, corporate or otherwise, to help them if they are struggling in any area, or alternatively to maintain the health of their business and help them to grow.

It bodes well for the success of a company, if both

management and employees are well balanced and happy in their work. The way energy works, is that it has a ripple effect. People that are happy at work, become happier at home. Parents that are happier at home, result in children that are happier and so it goes on. Within business, the ripples are just as profound, resulting in happier employees, better working conditions, improved sales, higher profits and so on and so forth. If management is happy, then so is the workforce.

Choose. Choose to make your workplace a happy place by healing the energies within your business.

About Yvette K Smith

Yvette began her career in the corporate world but became an entrepreneur once she had children and became a stay-at-home mother.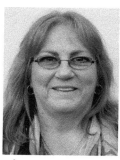

She has always been an inspiration and a mentor to others, which led her into a journey of discovery about energy medicine. After qualifying in this field, she now runs a successful practice in energy healing, which incorporates inspirational and success coaching.

Besides her busy life, Yvette has spent a significant amount of time helping in non-profit organisations like The Women's Institute and the Rotary Anns. She has also provided energy healing services to care homes and hospices.

She has been happily married for 41 years and is mother to three wonderful children; and a grandmother of one.

Yvette is a published author and currently lives in London.

Contact Yvette K Smith

ukbodytalk4health@gmail.com

Linked In: Yvette Smith, BodyTalk Practitioner (CBP)

https://www.linkedin.com/in/yvette-smith-bodytalk-practitioner-cbp-34661134/

Blog: https//energymatters.siterubix.com/

I Am Gratitude

Hana Abdelkhalek

It all began in March 2019. The pandemic hit Asia and contaminated Mother Earth. And I discovered meditation. To me meditation was a new concept, which I thought meant idolising a statue, which is forbidden in Islam.

One night, I was keen to learn more about meditation and the Universe put me in touch with Jasmine who had been meditating for six months. She had spoken before about meditation, but I wasn't ready at that time to understand and discover this beautiful aspect of our inner world. I remember that night, we had just finished a workout in the gym, and I asked her, *What is meditation? How do you meditate?* I had a lot of questions and was ashamed at the same time. Jasmine was delighted that I finally wanted to know more about that fabulous world.

That night, she gave me the Instagram profile of an uplifting meditation coach Medhi Selmi so that I could attend daily complimentary meditation sessions that were being held during quarantine to ease, lighten and brighten the negative effects of the overwhelming stress that was being endured by all human beings. And so, my journey began.

I remember my first meditation, as if it were yesterday. I was lying on my bed, it was an overwhelming experience. At a certain point my whole body shivered as if it was bathing in icy water. Being so new to meditation, I sent a message to the coach and explained what had happened and he suggested I cover myself with a light blanket. I then tried the technique of imagining my breath being sent to different parts of the body and I felt lighter, calmer, and more at peace. It was a fabulous experience because my body needed an opportunity to not only be able to relax and rest freely without any tension; but also to sink into my bed and have a deep, soothing sleep. What a powerful state of being I had been introduced to!

As a result, I continued attending online live meditations. One day, nearly at the end of a session, we were encouraged to put our hands on our hearts and thank God (or the Universe, the Super Power or Intelligence that rules the universe) and be grateful for the moment. For the first time in my life, I felt something like a spinning vortex around my heart, an overwhelming feeling and a weird sensation in and around my heart that made me cry. I felt as if I was hugging and squeezing my heart in my arms and hands. What an incredible experience!

That unprecedented, unrivalled feeling and rush of emotions triggered a mind-blowing, heartwarming sensation that shook me to my core and made me speechless for some time. I realized the existence of hidden powers, feelings, emotions that need to be unraveled to discover the tremendous beauty and the hidden power of our feelings.

And that moment, I understood the importance of gratitude. I began implementing gratitude whenever it was possible - during my morning routines, whilst alone, jogging, taking a walk in nature...

Gratitude is now as much a part of my daily life, just as breathing is. Expressing gratitude is so easy. Just begin with the two most powerful words in the English language: *I am...* and add positive uplifting words to feel, live and really believe what comes next. It could even be: *I am gratitude, I am Love, I am health.*

Your gratitude could also form a longer sentence, such as: *I am grateful for....* You can choose whatever best suits and reflects your best thinking in that moment.

I realised that I am grateful for every single part of my life. I am stepping out of my comfort zone, getting rid of those limiting beliefs and wholeheartedly tapping into my Best Life. I feel, and I believe that by nurturing my gratitude and using such powerful statements that my confidence has been boosted, and I have unleashed my potential to walk tall.

This attitude of gratitude is allowing me to reach for the stars. Dr John Demartini said that from the age of four, his mother encouraged him to count his blessings. I was conscious that if this helped him become the #1 world renowned Human Behavioural Specialist that it is achievable for me and every single person willing to elevate their lives to the next level.

As a result of exploring this marvellous inner world, and by willingly implementing these powerful gratitude incantations, I am seeing evidence that every tiny cell in my body has responded and I am now living congruent with how I am supposed to be living.

The gratitude blueprint is now a non-negotiable part of my morning routine. I am grateful for being introduced to gratitude.

It was a summer day in Tunisia. Instead of taking a taxi,

I walked feeling the connectedness to the trees, the singing birds, the gentle breeze, the fragrance of jasmine. When I met people in my neighbourhood I greeted them with a smile. I set the intention to respect the Earth, protect the environment and decrease pollution.

I now send my love through gratitude to everything I see, hear or smell. *I am grateful for all my senses.*

Out walking one day, I began saying things like: I am grateful for my nose to let me breathe in – breathe out the scented fragrance. I am grateful for my eyes, my clothes, my feelings, my health, my peace with myself.

Some seconds later, I was crying. I knew that slow conscious breathing slows and eases one's state of being, so I applied what I knew. You are fine, Hana. All is well. All is well is a powerful and mantra from Abraham Hicks. It eases one's state of being.

I stopped crying and smiled and even laughed – many mixed feelings were processed at the same time. Then I went through my gratitude process, since it is a non-negotiable part of my morning routine. I cried again and did conscious breathing to experience and elevate a genuine feeling of gratitude. James McNeil says: Gratitude is the attitude for altitude.

I relived that moment again and again until I reached work that day. The tears were just blissful to transcend and ignite a positive state of awareness, releasing the unconditional love inside of me.

I am grateful for unconditional Love.

After attending an online meditation workshop with my Best Life MBA community, my coach, JP, advised us to go outside to move our bodies: run, march, go jogging, connect with nature. I chose to go to a beach close by. I am convinced the human spirit needs time in nature so that we can appreciate being in the moment and be fully grounded. I walked along the beach, consciously breathing in the refreshing, calming sea air, greeting everyone with a big smile on my face, and of course practicing gratitude throughout. *I am grateful for my English skills. I am grateful for living my Best Life.*

I found a beautiful place with big yellow rocks on the shore and sat between them. I rested my back on one of those rocks, breathed deeply and started saying: I am Love concentrating on the breathtaking scenery of the endless sea. As I was repeating this affirmation, feeling the three little words... believing them... living them and saying them slower and slower, my body started tingling. I felt a warmth and goose bumps in my body from head to toes and suddenly and unexpectedly, cried. As I sat on that rock,

I really believed that I am Love.

I can't articulate enough the wonderful impact that these recently discovered little gems have had on me. I now live in a higher vibrational state of being. My heart seems wrapped with a positive, powerful, rewarding energy. It infuses every cell of my body. I feel compelled to sing about the magical effect of this higher vibrational state that shifts my whole being to a more profound state of consciousness as I connect to the hidden powers of Love - love that I have now for every sentient being.

These incredible feelings had been dormant inside of me waiting to be discovered and unravelled. Transcending to a higher vibrational state through the power of meditation is something that I continue to explore and have loved implementing into my life.

About Hana Abdelkhalek

Hana is a kind, compassionate, heart-centered, teacher who has worked in education for over 15 years. She applies best educational practices with love and compassion. Hana currently teaches children aged from 4 to 12.

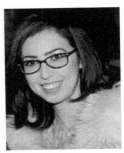

Hana is a CELTA qualified teacher and TA at the British Council Tunisia which has enabled her to further develop and uplevel her teaching skills.

Hana speaks four languages and enjoys the mental stimulation each language brings and enjoys the depth that language brings to the mental, physical and spiritual aspects of life.

Hana enjoys education, inner personal growth, auto healings and the healing power of plants. She wants to take her spirituality to the next level in order to understand more about herself and others. Hana is helping women through her interest in natural medicine and her ambition is to see those in her country able to access effective medicine and medical support.

Contact Hana Abdelkhalek

https://www.facebook.com/hana.abdelkhalek

https://www.instagram.com/hinnou/

In My Own Words

Kate McNeilly

Words come easy to me and I've loved my life to date and want to live fully until I die, making the world a better place before I pass on - and I've always longed for peace and I have always seen education as the Master Key with (lately) Gratitude as the Golden Key because that one opens hearts.

I could have titled this article *This World Is Not My Home, Finish Strong* or even *Full Circle* because I have been a conduit. I decided on the above because in a heartbeat, things can and do happen that change lives.

Professor Yuval Noah Hariri said in *Sapiens* when man developed language, he made giant leaps forward in connecting and communicating, separating from other species. It was speech that enabled the evolution of mankind.

A gifted teacher James Ramsey (Cambridge double first with a photographic memory) - opened this defiant teenage up to English and education, if not in a heartbeat then a few short months through language and experiences where I've been learning and sharing ever since.

My shorthand teacher, Emily Smith, shared a priceless tool which opened me up. In my mind's eye I can see in shorthand, I can feel it and I definitely need to hear it. Yes, I smell the ink and yes, I taste the words to see that they are good. Which led me to my sixth sense, intuition and spirituality. Using all of my senses, I've lived a sensual life. (Shorthand helps with enunciation and pronunciation but plays havoc with spelling because it is phonetic. Sir Isaac Pitman was a genius. Just as much as Einstein, Tesla and many other men and women).

How long does it take to become elite, sculpting your mind, body and spirit - your life? Ten thousand hours? Nay, a lifetime - and one lifetime is not enough. For all the geniuses who've ever lived and shared their art and science and all who have gone before us, thank you.

My first HUGE stretch goal was decided at 13 when I knew I wanted to work for the UN because I'm a pacifist at heart. I had 4 brothers then and felt

I would lose them to war because they were fit and healthy and would be conscripted. I knew I would do my bit for peace. My "great" uncle, Mr R R Bowman talked about the work of the UN, opening up a whole new world, when he asked, 'What do you want to do with your life, young lady'.

I knew in a heartbeat. I passed my medical in Harley Street and was accepted to work for the UN in Geneva. Once accepted, again instantly, I decided instead to stay in London. It was late 1960s! I've no regrets, having come full circle.

I've been book editing for 40 years, amongst other things, preserving the best and discarding the rest. What a phenomenal world we live in, even more than ever and what a beautiful world it will be when we have peace. JP endeared himself to me when I saw his wrist band *Peace and Unity*. I saw that in a heartbeat. I have his second wristband too, *I'm Extraordinary*, which we all are, and I know there's nothing ordinary about us. As the Bible says:"In an awe-inspiring way I'm wonderfully made" - Psalms 139:4.

Not just words, life too needs editing and auditing, as we find less truly is more. It helps to have an elite coach in different areas requiring focus. For me right now, health and wealth are vital.

We've finally reached a point where we can see starkly what lies ahead. This clarity means that we need to take time to adjust our paths towards peace and unity - and to finish strong, as JP says. Recognising all the while that the earth does not belong to us, we are caretakers, and we are all one race, the human race.

More than ever in 2020, it's tough to embrace the future when you are still focused on the past - so let go of your stories and get in the game of life. Get a coach or two and be in community, no masking.

It's a case of Mind, Body, Spirt and the biggest changes in my life have been when I fully grasped and experienced the spiritual aspects of life - particularly after a near death accident in 2015, two hours to curtains, when

I was mowed down outside my driveway by a delivery driver. My near death experience (NDE) was seeing and hearing my mother speak in my mind's eye (under the influence of morphine perhaps) when I saw four deceased members of my family clear as day, mother, father, Joan my eldest sister and niece Julie overlooking me with Mummy saying, *"Come on Kate, you can do this"*.

I knew in a heartbeat that I would recover from my accident and trauma. Trauma, what trauma? I found out in hospital on 28 October 2015. It was a wake up call, same as two awful times before in my life – my niece Julie's murder at the age of 5 ½ by a paedophile; my nephew Gareth losing most his right leg in a motorbike accident (first microprocessor leg in the UK and he went on win the Phoenix Cup for disabled golfers (similar to the Ryder Cup) in October 2018 in Florida). And then my own accident which changed my life. My surgeon had to explain what a pulmonary embolism is and - awaiting a fifth operation - I'm still healing.

Trauma is a process and there are more tools now to deal with it than then. I've discovered that many things to do with growth and learning are processes. I couldn't talk about Julie's abduction and murder for 30 years and rarely mentioned it until an opportunity at Toastmasters when the murderer was let out of prison on parole. Three judges who sentenced him all said life but they died and he appealed. I found I had to process all that.

London is my base. It truly is a world city with unique energy. Every day I need to fill my lungs and be in nature. But when I need more air and sunshine, I travel. Now we have AirBnB and technology I'm ready to go once restrictions are lifted. In the meantime, peace and education are non-negotiables for me.

Eighteen months ago, I went solo to Australia for six glorious weeks, with a stick, holdall bag and iPhone. Australia reminded me of the red earth of Africa which gets in your soul as experienced in South Africa, Zambia and Zaire in the 1980s. Same with America starting in 1984. All vast continents, not countries. In any event, the earth does not belong to us, we're just a-passing through. I'm no longer interested in nationalities, divisions, no country getting on with its neighbours. We recognise a tree by the fruitage it produces, same with politics and religion for me.

I've had a rich, varied life, living in London, travelling the world, but I was in a hurry going nowhere, at the time of my accident. Two hours to curtains, what a wake up call. Now I know where I'm going. I'm just a-passing through this beautiful earth, fitter and happier than I've ever been - and I still want to make a difference, peace through education has always been my focus. I teach, mentor and coach, so I've touched the future as mine has been touched by the people I've met, the books I've read and so much more.

Health is a lifestyle that includes mind, body and spirit and I've learnt much through BLMBA, from deep nutrition, breathwork, meditation and through the many speakers and experts JP has introduced, just like Tony Robbins before him.

All the holy books, all religions espouse love and truth and I would rather see a sermon than hear one. I believe we're 100% human, 100% divine. But sometimes only death reminds us we are alive.

Full of cliches and mixed metaphors, I know, because many before me have had similar experiences.

An all-time favourite book, Sensual Home by Ilse Crawford, an architect, talks about liberating your senses to change your life – and she's right. Key words are harmony, balance, peace, comfort, texture, space, proportion, energy, spirit, light, shade, sustenance – and love. If a book contains one golden nugget, a paragraph, it's worth the price – and I'm very selective about what I let into my mind and heart now.

Writing is another stretch goal for me, to step out from behind, not just editing. This is the first time I'm writing as me and not transcribing other's words. It won't be the last. And I shall continue to use modern technology to communicate and connect. I am a nurturer, never married because of my niece Julie's murder by a paedophile in July 1981, and I know I am a fierce mother tiger. An aside, I couldn't bear the thought of bringing children into a world where awful things happen and believed that no man would want to marry me because I didn't want children. So, it was heads down as I worked in the City top level for 40 years, mainly in banking, law and education, with community work evenings and weekends. I care little about the opinions of others because I'm living my one wild, precious life, my best life. I have the confidence now. And if not now, then when?

I've learnt how to speak in public, be on radio and video. I knew I had to find my voice, which is why I joined Toastmasters in 2001 and became a Distinguished Toastmaster (DTM), being actively involved in setting up 14 clubs in London, mentoring hundreds from all over the world over the years, all gratis. That's where I learnt to lead because I've been brought up to raise my head above the parapet if no one else does. Generations of women before me did. And it's been a joy to watch others progress and prosper. Ask me about the Julie Technique, a brief talk I gave at Toastmasters years ago, about getting in first! And here I am - almost last in the book - finishing strong, in a stream of awakened consciousness.

This is my second chance, and by golly I'm taking it - so time to ditch outdated beliefs and seize opportunities by releasing control and aligning my life to the divine within. Simple but not easy for most because of culture and conditioning. So, let's live on purpose, let's make peace a reality through education, and let's make a difference.

About Kate McNeilly

Kate McNeilly was the world's fastest shorthand writer (300 wpm), used in court rooms and boardrooms throughout the world.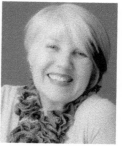

She mastered many skills in news, law, banking, academia and technology.

She is a Master of NLP and a Colour and Image Consultant, as her passion is colour and her home is her studio.

She is Co-Founder of London Athenians & West London Speakers Toastmasters' clubs and was deeply involved in setting up 14 others in and around London.

She lives in London which she uses as a base to travel the world, educating herself and others.

Only So Many Tomorrows is the quote that kept Kate alive during rehabilitation four and a half years ago. It is the title of her forthcoming book that will be available on Amazon soon.

Contact Kate McNeilly

https://www.facebook.com/katemcneilly

www.linkedin.com/in/Kate-McNeilly-0103

Instagram: @katie_47mac

Unlocking Your Best Life

Andrew Priestley Grad Dip Psych, B.Ed

I hope you are enjoying the stories in *Your Best Life*. This article is designed to help you get even more from this book by discovering and understanding the change strategies embedded in the stories, and then perhaps better applying it to your story.

In each story, the authors are either describing a change in a *specific situation* they were struggling with ie., conflict, confidence; a *specific life area* i.e., relationships, health, finances; or a *wholesale global transformation* i.e., addict to athlete.

The authors describe *transitioning* from State A (a specific current situation or set of circumstances) to State B (a more positive and healthy situation or set of circumstances).

In all the stories, the journey for State A to B typically describes overcoming limitations or obstacles. The limitations are either *real* (skills, behaviours, competencies, barriers); *self imposed* (attitudes, beliefs); or a combination of those two.

The reason they lock in those desired changes reflects *transformation* - a change in beliefs, attitudes, mindset, inspiration etc. Supercoach Michael Neil (2009) describes transformation as a change on the inside whilst maintaining a forward momentum towards external goals.

We can observe that in each story they need to *stop* doing something that isn't working; *start* doing something better that does work; *continue* doing what works; and of course, review progress.

When I mentor business leaders, I pay close attention to how they describe their current challenges; and how they future pace the changes they need to make. I notice especially how they explain why something did or didn't work.

The key is language patterns.

Someone I admire greatly is   Dr Robert Dilts, who contributed research to neuro-linguistic programming (NLP); importantly language patterns for shifting beliefs.

Dilts asked, *Why are some changes so much easier to achieve than others? And once achieved, why do some last … and some don't?*

He proposed that whether on a personal or organisational level, logically, it's all to do with the level on which you're trying to make the change.

Dilts defined six levels that influence how you think about a situation: *environment, behaviour; skills* (capability/ competence); *beliefs* (values); *identity;* and *intention* (greater purpose/ spirituality).

Recognising that a problem might be occurring at one or more levels gives you a helpful structure for unpacking each of the stories in this book; and a better way to understand your own challenges.

Environment (Where, When With Whom?)

Environment or circumstances is about external conditions. When the author is explaining what happened, when, who and so on, they are explaining what happened to them.

For example, I was minding my own business and a pandemic happened. The stock market crashed. The Global Financial Crisis occurred. The people at work are mean to me … the kids at school are bullies … I got ill, I was married to a sociopathic, narcissist etc.

The story is about what happened *outside of them*. And you will hear about how people and situations - circumstances - impacted their life and may be even responsible for why their problems.

Listen out for *where, when, with whom*. And see if you are naturally thinking: *What happened …? And then what?*

Behaviour (What?)

Behaviour is actions and reactions by an individual to *what's* occurring within that environment or set of circumstances. At this level you will hear them describing *what* they did, said or thought; and *what* effect that had or didn't have. It can also include *what* they might have done, could have done, should have done; and *what* effect that might have had.

In coaching we use a technique called *Reset the clock to zero*. We ask the client to describe *what* they might have done differently. Or what they might do differently... next time. Essentially, this is revising the situation or circumstances using a more empowering narrative.

Listen out for *what. What did you do? What (behaviour) do you need to do?*

Skills (How?)

Skills cover capabilities, competencies, knowledge, experiences and relates to *how* something was done; or not done. Skills or the lack of shape what you do - your behaviour - which impacts the circumstances. At this level, they are describing how to achieve something, or reflecting on the skills you might need to achieve the changes you prefer.

Listen out for *how*. How did you do that ...?

Beliefs/Values (Why?)

Belief is usually about *why* something can or can't occur. It often is influenced by underlying values. Beliefs and values reinforce or undermine skill acquisition (how you do it) ... which influence behaviour (what you do) ... which impact circumstances. For example, a belief that you are stuck could undermine any attempt to extricate yourself from a situation you don't like, i.e., I can't leave my job.

When working with clients I might ask, *Why did this happen?* I'm listening for their *explanatory style*.

If you read JP's story you can see a empowering explanatory style at work that allowed him to cope with an horrific hit and run accident, that was not his fault, which he accepted responsibility for, anyway, as a masterful way of coping.

Notice Simon swam the English Channel because he had the skills but the belief that he could. (And the intention to raise money for charity.)

Notice Angela's parting comments about her new empowering identity... and how it is held in place by resourceful beliefs.

Notice how Alison has reframed her identity to athlete supported by empowering new skills and behaviours and an intention to live a life she has chosen.

Listen out for *why* (I can or can't, or must or must not, or have to etc.)

Identity (Who?)

Identity is about *who* you are. Self-concept. Your sense of self. Typically, people will say *I am* or *I am not*, i.e., *I am stuck, I am not good enough. I am good with money. I am a good cook. I am not a good cook.*

I am an imposter and I have imposter syndrome is an identity issue usually held in place by strong or confused disempowering beliefs. *I always sabotage my success. I always find some way to mess things up. I can't find a nice partner because I am not good enough.* Can you see how identity is the key issue here?

When you're reading the stories listen out for *I am/am not* statements. Or statements that infer that. You will recognise that a gear change at the identity level was critical to the change occurring.

Intention (What's the purpose?)

Purpose/intention is about a *bigger why?* JP does a lot of coaching around intention and a bigger purpose. Many of the authors mention being transformed by embracing a physical challenge. A stretch goal. You may have noticed the authors are throwing out this term *non-negotiable*. Both are about intention. Intention informs identity, belief, skill, behaviour and circumstances.

Clinically, we accept that all behaviour is purposeful. However, sometimes you do inappropriate or unresourceful things. Have you noticed? When that occurs, it flags that there's a *secondary gain* to a holding onto a non optimum situation, especially when it doesn't make any sense.

If I am working with a client I am asking, *What do you imagine is the purpose or intention for this identity ... or belief ... or skill ... or behaviour or circumstances? What purpose does it serve?*

You will recognise that each author asked, *What do I want? What needs to be better? What needs to be even better? What does good look like here for everyone?* It is inferred in any case.

Listen out for *Why I do what I do?* Ask yourself, whatever you are doing, saying or being - *what's the purpose?*

OK, with practice you can now figure out how someone changed, specifically, *where* it changed meaning at what level change occurred or was needed, just by carefully reading the story and noticing the language they use to describe what happened.

Dilts makes a lot of important observations but two that I find relevant.

First, it's harder to initiate change at the level you feel most stuck. If you feel blocked or stuck or helpless your problem or situation will seem unsolvable.

For example, if improving your life depends on someone else changing or being different you will probably wait along time. This dynamic underpins co-dependent relationships. Dilts suggests that change needs to occur at a different level to the level where you are most stuck.

Let's pretend you say, *Businesses today need to use social media to succeed. I'm no good at using Instagram, therefore, you cannot hold me responsible for the under performance of my business.* That example contains just about every level we have mentioned above.

I wonder if you can unpack it?

For example, *I believe I need to put my prices up, but I don't believe I am worth it. I will put my prices up when I believe I am worth it.* Where is this person stuck? The most?

Gavin was pummelled into a financial hole by the Global Financial Crisis (circumstances) but how did he claw his way back from those challenges? Notice his later insight about being responsible. What did he change? Importantly, *where* did he change? (Which level?) (Note: it may not have been deliberate. Dilts gives you a useful resource to make deliberate changes.

You will notice that each author had to change their focus to a different level than the one they were stuck in regardless of whether that was conscious or not. Only then the problem started to resolve. And they started to change.

Please note this tool does not guarantee rapid change, but it can give you a structure for making positive healthy changes, albeit incrementally.

If you have an issue, try changing your focus to another level. This will bring a new perspective. This is one of the tools JP often uses to help his MBA clients to think through problems. Tony Robbins does exactly this.

If you've tried to succeed at something and it's a struggle, then looking at the neurological levels can at least make things clearer.

If you want your circumstances to change:

Do you need to change your behaviours?

Do you need to develop (and practice) new skills?

Do you need to change your beliefs? You might not need to explore why do you believe you can or can't do something. Just recognising - *Ahhh, thats a belief!* - will start to unstick your stickiness, if that's even a word.

Spend time at the belief level and explore the secondary gain of staying stuck or helpless. Maybe it's a secret way that you get attention. Think of Lou and Andy from *Little Britain*.

Do you need to change your self-concept? Pay close attention to *I am/I am not* statements. *I am no good at public speaking* actually means you lack *skill* development and practice (behaviour). It doesn't mean you can't develop those skills. Ask Helen Keller.

If it is possible that you could develop those skills, but won't, then we need to - you need to, actually dig deeper.

Understand this is a very basic introduction to Dilts' model. I am very sure it may not be technically correct. But it's a start. I wanted to give you a useful lens for exploring how the authors made changes in *Your Best Life*. You have 21 stories to play around with.

If you do the work, the stories will make a lot more sense. You will see the way change happened, you'll hear your own *ah-ha* thoughts and insights, and you will be able to grab onto the value and run with it.

I hope this helps.

References

- Dilts, R. (1990). Changing Belief Systems With NLP, Meta Publications.

- Neil, M. (2009). Supercoach. Hayhouse

- https://www.skillsyouneed.com/lead/logical-levels.html

- Seligman. M, Ph.D. (1998). Learned Optimism. Simon & Schuster.

About Andrew Priestley

Andrew Priestley is an award-winning business leadership mentor qualified in Industrial and Organisational Psychology and ranked in the top 100 UK Mentors (2017). He is a bestselling author and in-demand speaker.

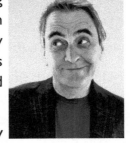

He is the Chairman of Clear Sky Children's Charity UK that provides play therapy for children aged 4-12 who have witnessed or directly experienced a trauma. He is a strategic advisor to the Mahler Foundation and sits on several NXD boards.

He loves to draw and cook. And he loves his garden.

Contact Andrew on LinkedIn.

About Best Life MBA Community

It's difficult to succeed in the game of life if you're not a champion in personal leadership. This means to be spiritually, mentally, emotionally and physically fit.

Being life-fit means having extraordinary energy and a winning attitude, and requires winning strategies, guidance and mentoring.

In your *Best Life MBA* I will coach you on how to deploy the best habits for your life fitness, provide you with the most effective tools and exercises, connect you with the greatest teachers and advise you on the best winning strategies for your life.

I will support you in the most important areas of personal growth and leadership, giving you education, motivation, inspiration and so much more. You deserve to be fit healthy, wealthy and happy, and to feel like you're winning in every area of your life.

I've made it happen for myself and I've made it happen for thousands of other people. Now it's your turn. What are you waiting for?

Make the commitment take action, and let me help you reach the highest level of personal performance and fully own your life.

Your *Best Life MBA* is how you will make it happen.

Jean-Pierre De Villiers

Join Best Life MBA

www.jeanpierredevilliers.com/best-life-mba

Would You Like To Contribute
To Future Editions of Your Best Life?

Your Best Life is written by the members of the *Best Life MBA* community. If you would like to get involved in the next release of *Your Best Life*, then ...

Join Best Life MBA

www.jeanpierredevilliers.com/best-life-mba

Lightning Source UK Ltd.
Milton Keynes UK
UKHW010854171220
375409UK00003B/63